CSA
REVISION
NOTES
FOR THE
MRCGP

D0589539

ALSO OF INTEREST

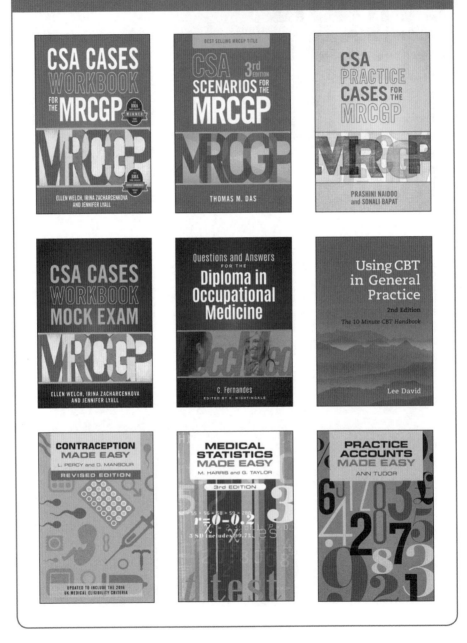

For more details see www.scionpublishing.com

Third Edition

CSA REVISION NOTES FOR THE MRCGP

Jennifer Stannett
BSc (Hons), MBChB, MRCGP, MRCPCH, DRCOG, DFSRH
GP in Bath

Sarah Osmond
MBChB, FRNZCGP
GP in Dumfriesshire

Scion

© **Scion Publishing Limited, 2016**

ISBN 978 1 907904 84 4

Third edition first published 2016

Second edition (ISBN 978 1 907904 07 3) published 2013

First edition published 2011

All rights reserved. No part of this book may be reproduced or transmitted, in any form or by any means, without permission.

A CIP catalogue record for this book is available from the British Library.

Scion Publishing Limited

The Old Hayloft, Vantage Business Park, Bloxham Road, Banbury OX16 9UX, UK

www.scionpublishing.com

Important Note from the Publisher

The information contained within this book was obtained by Scion Publishing Ltd from sources believed by us to be reliable. However, while every effort has been made to ensure its accuracy, no responsibility for loss or injury whatsoever occasioned to any person acting or refraining from action as a result of information contained herein can be accepted by the authors or publishers.

Readers are reminded that medicine is a constantly evolving science and while the authors and publishers have ensured that all dosages, applications and practices are based on current indications, there may be specific practices which differ between communities. You should always follow the guidelines laid down by the manufacturers of specific products and the relevant authorities in the country in which you are practising.

Although every effort has been made to ensure that all owners of copyright material have been acknowledged in this publication, we would be pleased to acknowledge in subsequent reprints or editions any omissions brought to our attention.

Registered names, trademarks, etc. used in this book, even when not marked as such, are not to be considered unprotected by law.

Typeset by Phoenix Photosetting, Chatham, Kent, UK

Printed in the UK

Contents

Contents

Contents

Preface to the third edition

This new updated edition is the result of both your helpful feedback and many hours spent researching the latest clinical evidence and national guidelines.

I am delighted that the previous editions have helped so many candidates in their exam preparation. I have therefore kept the basic format of the book the same. I have added a few new topics, which I felt would be useful to the reader, and updated existing topics.

The examination chapter has been updated as there have been many changes since the last edition.

As with the previous edition, I would encourage readers to use this book like a revision workbook in combination with seeing plenty of patients in the GP surgery.

I wish you the best of luck with the CSA exam and every success in general practice!

Jennifer Stannett
April 2016

About the authors

Jennifer Stannett gained a biomedical sciences degree from the University of Manchester before studying medicine at Leicester–Warwick Medical School. She spent two years working in paediatrics before completing vocational GP training in London. After spending a year travelling the world, she now works as a GP partner in Bath.

Sarah Osmond studied medicine at the University of Edinburgh. She then spent five years working in New Zealand where she completed her GP training. She now works as a GP partner and trainer in Dumfriesshire, Scotland.

Acknowledgements

Thanks to Paul Dakin for your help, advice and inspiration to get involved in medical writing.

Thanks to Sharon Stannett for your help with the book illustrations.

Most importantly, thanks to our families for being so supportive over the years and helping us to reach our goals.

Preface to the first edition

This book provides a summary of clinical cases which could be tested in the CSA exam, divided up into topics based on the MRCGP syllabus.

It aims to help prepare candidates for the CSA exam by providing a basic structure for consulting, focusing on the three key areas of data gathering, clinical management and interpersonal skills. The information is displayed in a concise manner in order to provide a quick reference guide for the candidate. It does not contain detailed clinical information. In the data gathering section, the most important aspects of history taking have been included and usually, but not always, cover history of the presenting complaint, past medical history, drug history, family history, and social history. Red flags have also been highlighted, where relevant, to act as a prompt to the reader to ask these important questions. Example questions have been included and these could be asked to explore the patient's ideas, concerns and expectations. I would also encourage you to think of your own alternative questions which you may also ask in the exam.

In the clinical management section I have included possible investigation and management options based on the latest UK guidelines. Not all options will be appropriate in every case, so it is important for the reader to consider each case individually.

Every case includes an explanation to the patient, which I hope will help the reader to think about how they would discuss each condition with the patient in jargon-free terms.

At the end of each case there is a role play scenario which can be practised in small groups or with a study partner. The information given to the doctor is similar to that which you will encounter in the CSA. The role player's brief should not be read by the doctor and so I suggest that the role player reads their information first and covers up the information (a Post-it note is ideal) before showing the doctor their information. Alternatively, the role player can read the brief to the doctor. The brief for the role player has deliberately been kept quite short in order to make it quick and easy to read, and the information in bold is that which should only be offered if asked about specifically by the doctor. Other clinical details can be added by the role player if necessary. The examination findings included in some cases can be given to the doctor if specifically requested, or alternatively they provide a good opportunity to practise these clinical examinations.

After completing each case in this book, it is important to reflect on how well you did in the role play scenario, and how you might improve your performance. It may be useful to ask the role player for their feedback. To make the most of the book, the role play scenarios should be practised under exam conditions. If working with a study partner, you could discuss each case in turn, teasing out various issues and then practising the scenarios again, trying out different techniques and consultation styles.

An explanation of the marking scheme and tips for success can be found in the first chapter, and the book concludes with appendices summarising the different clinical examinations which you could be expected to perform.

I would encourage readers to use this book like a workbook, gradually working through each clinical topic, and annotating it with your own aides-memoire to facilitate your learning. In the weeks leading up to the exam the book should be used in combination with lots of real patient consultations in the GP surgery. Together these will ensure that you go into the exam well prepared and confident.

Good luck!

Jennifer Stannett
December 2010

Abbreviations

A&E	Accident and emergency department	DRE	Digital rectal examination
		DSH	Deliberate self harm
ABPM	Ambulatory blood pressure monitoring	DVLA	Driver and Vehicle Licensing Agency
ACE	Angiotension converting enzyme	DVT	Deep vein thrombosis
ACR	Albumin creatinine ratio	ECG	Electrocardiogram
ADHD	Attention deficit hyperactivity disorder	ENT	Ear, nose and throat
		EPAU	Early pregnancy assessment unit
AF	Atrial fibrillation	ESR	Erythrocyte sedimentation rate
AFP	Alpha fetoprotein	FBC	Full blood count
ALP	Alkaline phosphatase	FEV1	Forced expiratory volume in 1 second
AMSE	Abbreviated mental state examination		
		FH	Family history
BMI	Body mass index	FP10	Blank prescription
BNF	*British National Formulary*	FSH	Follicle stimulating hormone
BP	Blood pressure	FVC	Forced vital capacity
CBT	Cognitive behavioural therapy	GFR	Glomerular filtration rate
CF	Cystic fibrosis	GGT	Gamma glutamyl transferase
CHD	Coronary heart disease	GI	Gastrointestinal
CK	Creatine kinase	GMC	General Medical Council
CKD	Chronic kidney disease	GnRH	Gonadotrophin releasing hormone
CKS	*Clinical Knowledge Summaries*	GORD	Gastro-oesophageal reflux disease
COCP	Combined oral contraceptive pill	GTN	Glyceryl trinitrate
COPD	Chronic obstructive pulmonary disease	GU	Genito-urinary
		Hb	Haemoglobin
CPAP	Continuous positive airways pressure	HbA1C	Glycosylated haemoglobin
		hCG	Human chorionic gonadotrophin
CRP	C-reactive protein	HDL	High density lipoprotein
CRT	Capillary refill time	HONK	Hyperosmolar non-ketosis
CT	Computerised tomography	HPA	Health Protection Agency
CVD	Cardiovascular disease	HPC	History of presenting complaint
CVS	Cardiovascular system	HRT	Hormone replacement therapy
CXR	Chest X-ray	IBD	Inflammatory bowel disease
D&V	Diarrhoea and vomiting	IBS	Irritable bowel syndrome
DEXA	Dual energy X-ray absorptiometry	ICE	Ideas, concerns and expectations
DH	Drug history	ICP	Intracranial pressure
DKA	Diabetic ketoacidosis	ICS	Inhaled corticosteroid
DM	Diabetes mellitus	IDDM	Insulin-dependent diabetes mellitus
DMARD	Disease-modifying antirheumatic drug		
		IMB	Intermenstrual bleeding
DoH	Department of Health	IRT	Immuno-reactive trypsinogen

IUCD	Intra-uterine contraceptive device		PMB	Post-menopausal bleeding
ITU	Intensive Therapy Unit		PMR	Polymyalgia rheumatica
IUD	Intra-uterine device		PMS	Pre-menstrual syndrome
IVDU	Intravenous drug user		PO	*Per os* (orally)
LABA	Long acting beta agonist		PPI	Proton pump inhibitor
LAMA	Long acting muscarinic agonist		PR	*Per rectum* (rectally)
LDH	Lactate dehydrogenase		PRN	As required
LDL	Low density lipoprotein		PSA	Prostate specific antigen
LFTs	Liver function tests		PTSD	Post-traumatic stress disorder
LMP	Last menstrual period		PV	*Per vaginum* (vaginally)
LNG-IUS	Levonorgestrel intra-uterine system		PVD	Peripheral vascular disease
			QDS	*Quarter die sumendus* (to be taken four times a day)
LVF	Left ventricular failure			
MC&S	Microscopy, culture and sensitivities		RA	Rheumatoid arthritis
			RhF	Rheumatoid factor
MED3	Fit for work certificate		RICE	Rest, ice, compression, elevation
MI	Myocardial infarction		ROM	Range of movement
MMSE	Mini mental state examination		RR	Respiratory rate
MRI	Magnetic resonance imaging		RUQ	Right upper quadrant
MSU	Mid-stream urine		SC	Sub-cutaneously
NAAT	Nucleic acid amplification test		SE	Side effect
NAD	No abnormalities detected		SH	Social history
NG	Naso-gastric		SHBG	Sex hormone binding globulin
NICE	National Institute for Health and Clinical Excellence		SL	Sublingual
			SOB	Shortness of breath
NIDDM	Non-insulin dependent diabetes mellitus		SSRI	Selective serotonin re-uptake inhibitor
NSAID	Non-steroidal anti-inflammatory drug		STI	Sexually transmitted infection
			SVT	Supraventricular tachycardia
NTDs	Neural tube defects		T3	Triiodothyronine
OA	Osteoarthritis		T4	Thyroxine
OD	*Omni die* (once daily)		TCC	Transitional cell carcinoma
O/E	On examination		TDS	*Ter die sumendus* (to be taken three times a day)
ON	*Omni nocte* (every night)			
ONS	Office of National Statistics		TFTs	Thyroid function tests
OSAS	Obstructive sleep apnoea syndrome		TIA	Transient ischaemic attack
			TOP	Termination of pregnancy
PALS	Patient Advice and Liaison Service		TSH	Thyroid stimulating hormone
PAPP-A	Pregnancy-associated plasma protein A		U&Es	Urea and electrolytes
			UI	Urinary incontinence
PCB	Post-coital bleeding		UPSI	Unprotected sexual intercourse
PCOS	Polycystic ovarian syndrome		USS	Ultrasound scan
PE	Pulmonary embolus		UTI	Urinary tract infection
PEFR	Peak expiratory flow rate		VT	Ventricular tachycardia
PHQ	Patient health questionnaire		VTE	Venous thromboembolism
PID	Pelvic inflammatory disease		2WW	Two week wait

Introduction to the CSA examination

The CSA examination is both a clinical and a consulting skills examination. It is one of three parts of the MRCGP, the other two being the Applied Knowledge Test (AKT) and the Workplace-Based Assessment (WPBA). The CSA is run three times a year and candidates can apply at any time during their GP registrar year. The CSA takes place in the Examination Centre at the RCGP's new headquarters at 30 Euston Square, London.

The CSA examination is defined by the RCGP as '*An assessment of a doctor's ability to integrate and apply appropriate clinical, professional, communication and practical skills in general practice.*' The exam is based on the RCGP curriculum, and the cases are selected to include the wide spectrum found in everyday general practice.

Format of the examination

The CSA examination consists of 13 consultations, each of 10 minutes' duration. The circuit takes approximately 3 hours to complete. All 13 cases will be marked.

Patients are played by trained and calibrated role players. Examiners are working GPs who are selected, trained and monitored to sit in, observe and mark each candidate. There will be a different examiner for each case, with the examiner always remaining with the same role player and case for the entire duration. The examiner will play no part in the consultation, except possibly to pass on information/results of examinations at appropriate points. They will sit outside your line of vision, and you should ignore them. It is possible that an additional observer may be present; they may be performing a Quality Assurance exercise or merely observing the process. They will take no part in your examination.

Candidates stay in the same consulting room throughout the whole examination, the only exception being for a home visit or telephone consultation case.

A mounted iPad will be available on the consulting desk with a patient list displayed. Information on how to access patient notes via this device will be given at a briefing session prior to commencing the exam. There are a few minutes to look through these notes prior to the examination starting. There are also 2 minutes between each case to look through these notes. The notes will include basic information about the patient, for example, name, age, relevant past medical history, current medication and social history. A wipe-clean A4 white board will be provided to make notes, although this won't be marked.

A buzzer sounds to mark the start and end of each case, and there is a 15 minute break at the end of the seventh case.

The role player will respond to your normal consultation style, although will not tell you their whole script unless you ask the appropriate questions. They will not, however, deliberately conceal vital information.

A clinical examination may be required, and the examination you choose and how this is performed will be marked. You will not be expected to do any intimate examinations.

Mock prescriptions and Med3 sickness certificates can also be given to the role player, and these may be marked. These will be provided on the desks.

Candidates can offer patient information leaflets to patients, and can ask the patient to collect these from reception after the consultation. It is important to explain briefly the content of the information leaflet in order to gain credit for this.

If the consultation comes to a natural end before 10 minutes, the patient and examiner will get up and leave. Alternatively, if you haven't finished your consultation by the time the buzzer sounds at the end of 10 minutes, the patient and examiner will leave and you will not be marked for anything which happens after the buzzer.

Candidates are required to take a limited amount of equipment to the exam, including both a BNF and a children's BNF which can be used for reference during the examination. Further guidance on what to bring can be found on the RCGP website. Other equipment, for example growth charts, peak flow charts and an obstetric dial, is provided.

Marking scheme

Each of the thirteen cases is marked by a different trained examiner using a pre-set marking schedule which is specific to the case. The pass mark is set using a 'borderline group' method, which allows for day to day variability in the difficulty of case mixes. The examiner marks each case on three domains or areas:
- data gathering
- clinical management
- interpersonal skills

This creates an overall numerical mark for the case. Each domain carries the same number of marks. The marks for each case are added to create a final mark for all 13 cases. A pass mark will have been set by the combined judgements of the examiners for that day.

The CSA can only be attempted a maximum of four times. Results and feedback are given via ePortfolio.

The following points highlight the key skills being assessed in each of the three domains.

Data gathering
- Organised and systematic in gathering information from history taking, examination and investigation

- Able to identify abnormal findings or results and recognise their implications
- Able to undertake physical examination competently, or use instruments proficiently

Clinical management

- Able to make an appropriate diagnosis
- Able to develop a management plan (including prescribing and referral) that is appropriate and in line with current best practice
- Able to demonstrate an awareness of management of risk and health promotion

Interpersonal skills

- Able to identify patient's agenda, health beliefs and preferences / makes use of verbal and non-verbal cues
- Identifies or uses appropriate psychological or social information to place the problem in context
- Develops a shared management plan or clarifies the role of doctor and patient
- Uses explanations that are relevant and understandable to the patient
- Shows sensitivity for the patient's feelings in all aspects of the consultation including physical examination

As well as marking the domain scores, the examiners will also mark each case separately using one of four possible grades:

- clear pass
- pass
- fail
- clear fail

Further details of these grade descriptors can be found on the RCGP website.

The RCGP website should be regularly checked for updated advice about the exam marking schemes.

Data gathering

Positive indicators	Negative indicators
- Clarifies the problem and nature of decision required - Uses an incremental approach, using time and accepting uncertainty - Gathers information from history taking, examination and investigation in a systematic and efficient manner - Is appropriately selective in the choice of enquiries, examinations and investigations - Identifies abnormal findings or results and makes appropriate interpretations - Uses instruments appropriately and fluently - When using instruments or conducting physical examinations, performs actions in a rational sequence	- Makes immediate assumptions about the problem - Intervenes rather than using appropriate expectant management - Is disorganised/unsystematic in gathering information - Data gathering does not appear to be guided by the probabilities of disease - Fails to identify abnormal data or correctly interpret them - Appears unsure of how to operate/use instruments - Appears disorganised/unsystematic in the application of the instruments or the conduct of physical examinations

Clinical management

Positive indicators	Negative indicators
• Recognises presentations of common physical, psychological and social problems • Makes plans that reflect the natural history of common problems • Offers appropriate and feasible management options • Management approaches reflect an appropriate assessment of risk • Makes appropriate prescribing decisions • Refers appropriately and co-ordinates care with other healthcare professionals • Manages risk effectively, safety netting appropriately • Simultaneously manages multiple health problems, both acute and chronic • Encourages improvement, rehabilitation, and, where appropriate, recovery • Encourages the patient to participate in appropriate health promotion and disease prevention strategies	• Fails to consider common conditions in the differential diagnosis • Does not suggest how the problem might develop or resolve • Fails to make the patient aware of relative risks of different approaches • Decisions on whether/what to prescribe are inappropriate or idiosyncratic • Decisions on whether and where to refer are inappropriate • Follow-up arrangements are absent or disjointed • Fails to take account of related issues or of co-morbidity • Unable to construct a problem list and prioritise • Unable to enhance patient's health perceptions and coping strategies

Interpersonal skills

Positive indicators	Negative indicators
• Explores patient's agenda, health beliefs and preferences • Appears alert to verbal and non-verbal cues • Explores the impact of the illness on the patient's life • Elicits psychological and social information to place the patient's problem in context • Works in partnership, finding common ground to develop a shared management plan • Communicates risk effectively to patients • Shows responsiveness to the patient's preferences, feelings and expectations • Enhances patient autonomy • Provides explanations that are relevant and understandable to the patient • Responds to needs and concerns with interest and understanding • Has a positive attitude when dealing with problems, admits mistakes and shows commitment to improvement • Backs own judgement appropriately • Demonstrates respect for others • Does not allow own views/values to inappropriately influence dialogue • Shows commitment to equality of care for all • Acts in an open, non-judgemental manner • Is cooperative and inclusive in approach • Conducts examinations with sensitivity for the patient's feelings, seeking consent where appropriate	• Does not inquire sufficiently about the patient's perspective/health understanding • Pays insufficient attention to the patient's verbal and nonverbal communication • Fails to explore how the patient's life is affected by the problem • Does not appreciate the impact of the patient's psychosocial context • Instructs the patient rather than seeking common ground • Uses a rigid approach to consulting that fails to be sufficiently responsive to the patient's contribution • Fails to empower the patient or encourage self-sufficiency • Uses inappropriate (e.g. technical) language • Shows little visible interest/understanding, lacks warmth in voice/manner • Avoids taking responsibility for errors • Does not show sufficient respect for others • Inappropriately influences patient interaction through own views/values • Treats issues as problems rather than challenges • Displays inappropriate favour or prejudice • Is quick to judge • Appears patronising or inappropriately paternalistic • When conducting examinations, appears unprofessional and at risk of hurting or embarrassing the patient

After the CSA exam, you will be informed of your performance overall and your grades for the thirteen cases. This is the 'summative' part of the feedback. In addition, you will also receive 'formative' feedback, which is designed to help you to reflect on possible areas for improvement.

Formative feedback is given in relation to 16 areas of performance (see below). Not all of these are tested in every consultation although they will be tested across the assessment as a whole. Any area of performance identified as deficient by two or more examiners will be flagged in feedback as an area for improvement.

The following are the main feedback statements (see the RCGP website for further information).

Global

1. Disorganised / unstructured consultation.
2. Does not recognise the issues or priorities in the consultation (for example, the patient's problem, ethical dilemma, etc.).
3. Shows poor time management.

Data gathering

4. Does not identify abnormal findings or results or fails to recognise their implications.
5. Does not undertake physical examination competently, or use instruments proficiently.

Clinical management

6. Does not make the correct working diagnosis or identify an appropriate range of differential possibilities.
7. Does not develop a management plan (including prescribing and referral) reflecting knowledge of current best practice.
8. Does not make adequate arrangements for follow-up and safety netting.
9. Does not demonstrate an awareness of management of risk or make the patient aware of relative risks of different options.
10. Does not attempt to promote good health at opportune times in the consultation.

Interpersonal skills

11. Does not appear to develop rapport or show sensitivity for the patient's feelings.
12. Does not identify or explore information about patient's agenda, health beliefs and preferences.
13. Does not make adequate use of verbal and non-verbal cues. Poor active listening skills.
14. Does not identify or use appropriate psychological or social information to place the problem in context.
15. Does not develop a shared management plan, demonstrating an ability to work in partnership with the patient.
16. Does not use language and/or explanations that are relevant and understandable to the patient.

Tips for success

Below are a few tips to help you get through the CSA examination.

Preparing for the CSA

- Practise 10 minute consultations in readiness for the exam.
- Have a timed structure to your consultations, for example, 5 minutes for history taking, 2–3 minutes for examination, and 2–3 minutes for clinical management.

- Keep a logbook of the cases that you see in the GP surgery, and read up on clinical details you are unsure about.
- Try joint surgeries with your trainer and video your consultations, as this is a great way to get constructive feedback.
- Focus on practising cases you are less confident with; for example, a female registrar may not feel too confident with an erectile dysfunction case!
- Practise your examination skills on friends or family, especially those examinations that you might not perform frequently.
- Make sure you can interpret common results such as ECGs and spirometry.
- Try to attend a CSA course beforehand as it can be a great confidence booster.

On the exam day

- Arrive early.
- Remember to bring all the necessary equipment.
- Use the alcohol gel provided in between patients.
- Read through any information provided before each case commences and make notes if necessary.
- You may find it helpful to write an aide-memoire on the white board provided with the key steps in history taking and the consultation (e.g. history, red flags, diagnosis, investigations and management, follow-up/safety netting).
- Make sure you cover all three domains within 10 minutes, as omission of any of these will result in a fail in that case.
- Be courteous and respectful towards the patients.
- Involve patients in decision making.
- Ensure that your explanations to patients are clear and jargon free.
- Drawing diagrams can be useful in aiding patient understanding.
- If you are referring a patient for further investigations or to secondary care, explain clearly what you intend to do.
- Check the patient's understanding and ask if they have any questions.
- If you lose your train of thought, try summarising the information you have already collected.
- If you feel one case didn't go so well, try to forget about it and regain your composure for future cases – remember you can still pass overall even if you fail some cases.
- Remember good communication skills and adopt a patient-centred approach.
- Try to remain calm.

General practice consultation

Telephone consultation

- In a climate of increasing targets and demand for access, telephone consultations are playing an increasingly important role in the delivery of healthcare by GPs.
- The scope of telephone consultations is wide ranging, and includes management of acute and chronic problems, medication reviews, follow-up care and delivery of information.
- It is important to be aware of the limitations of telephone consultations. Telephone advice is not always appropriate, and they do not provide the non-verbal cues that make up around 50% of face to face consultations (*GPOnline*, 2008, *Consultation skills – telephone consultations*).
- Key skills in telephone consultations include active listening, frequent clarification and picking up cues such as changes in the tone of voice.

Framework for telephone consultations

Preparation
- Look through the patient's notes prior to the telephone call, familiarising yourself with their past medical history, medication history and recent consultations, etc.
- Have a notepad or paper available in case you need to take notes during the consultation.

Introduction
- Introduce yourself and ensure that you are speaking to the correct person to ensure confidentiality.
- Try to build a rapport through the tone of your voice.

Data gathering
- A detailed history is essential in the absence of physical examination and signs.
- Use open and focused/closed questions to include/exclude relevant conditions.
- Remember to exclude red flag symptoms.
- Establish what the patient is wanting from the telephone consultation, e.g. are they looking for telephone advice, investigations, emotional support, a home visit or even a GP appointment?
- Establish whether the patient needs to come in for a face-to-face assessment. If so, when?
- Does the patient have adequate support at home?

Summarising

- Ensure that you have established the patient's ideas, concerns and expectations.
- Allow time for the patient to ask questions.

Clinical management

- Agree on a plan of action and give clear information about when to seek further advice or help (safety net).
- Request that the patient repeats the advice given.
- Allow the patient to end the call first.

Documentation

- Accurate records should be kept for all telephone consultations, with details of the management plan and follow-up agreed with the patient.

Role play

Information for doctor	Additional information for role player
Patient: Master JA *Age*: 8 months *PMH*: Nil *DH*: Nil *Information*: Mrs A (JA's mother) contacted the surgery this morning for telephone advice as JA has had a fever. You are a locum GP.	*PC*: Fever since last night (39°C). Diarrhoea 6× since last night. Vomited 5× today. *HPC*: JA has not been eating or drinking much. Has been giving him regular Calpol. Loose stools but no blood. **Only 1 wet nappy today. Lethargic. Not as active. No rash.** *ICE*: **Mum worried as he is not keeping fluids down. Has been trying bottles of milk so far.** Would like him to be seen at the surgery.

Home visit

- Home visits remain an integral part of primary care, and are still regularly carried out by GPs.
- In 1995, 9% of all GP consultations in the UK were home visits, whereas in 2008 this had decreased to just 4% (ONS and DoH Survey).
- GPs tend to visit a patient at home when the patient is confined due to illness or disability, or when urgent treatment can be given more quickly by visiting.
- The disadvantage of a home visit is that it is very time consuming for the GP and there is not access to some medical equipment which might otherwise be available in the surgery.

Framework for home visit consultations

Preparation

- Ensure you read through the patient's notes prior to visiting, familiarizing yourself with the patient's past medical history, medication history, allergies and recent consultations. It is useful to take a print out of this information on a home visit.
- Ensure that you pack a doctors' bag with all the relevant equipment.

- Ring the patient beforehand to determine the reason for the home visit request and confirm with them that you will be visiting.
- To ensure your safety, let a member of staff know that you are going on a home visit and give the details of which patient you are visiting.

Data gathering

- Ask open questions, followed by focused questions including those to check for red flags.
- Establish social history: Is the patient coping at home? Is additional help required? Any safeguarding concerns?
- Examination.

Clinical management

- Decide if the patient is safe to remain at home or if they need to be referred to hospital.
- Are any further investigations required?
- Arrange community support, e.g. district nursing team, palliative care, if appropriate.
- Ask patient to repeat back information to check they have correctly understood.
- Ensure all the patient's concerns have been addressed.
- Is any medication required?
- Safety net – involve relative or partner in this conversation if appropriate.
- Clearly document the consultation when back at the surgery.

Role play

Information for doctor	Additional information for role player
Patient: Mrs JL *Age*: 90 years *SH*: Lives alone in a 1 bedroom ground floor flat. Has carers twice daily. *PMH*: COPD *DH*: Tiotropium 18 mcg 2 puffs daily; Seretide 250 mcg 1 puff twice daily *Information*: Patient's daughter phoned this morning requesting a visit for her mother as she has been increasingly breathless and not her usual self. She is also worried as she lives alone. You are a GP Registrar.	*PC*: "*I've had a bit of a cough over the past few days and can't walk very far without getting very breathless*". *PMH*: **Cough productive of green sputum. No haemoptysis.** Haven't been able to get out of the house. SOB on walking a few metres. **No chest pain. No fever. No vomiting. No rash.** *SH*: **Ex-smoker (gave up 15 yrs ago) – 40 pack year history.** *ICE*: "*I think my COPD is getting worse*". *O/E*: Temp 36.8°C. BP 120/70. HR 70, regular. No pallor. Heart sounds normal. Coarse crackles on right side of chest. Mild wheeze bilaterally.

Angry patient

- Managing an angry patient can be upsetting and potentially dangerous.
- The reason for a patient being angry can include anything from social or financial problems to difficulties getting GP appointments, poor communication, or a doctor ignoring their ideas, concerns and expectations.

- An angry patient can escalate to a violent patient. Signs of escalation include shouting, swearing, raising a clenched fist, pacing or adopting an aggressive posture.

Tips for managing an angry patient

- Remain professional and calm.
- Actively listen to the complaint.
- Find out specifically if there is anything they want you to do.
- Give the patient space and time to vent their anger.
- Apologise, for example by saying *"I'm sorry you've had to go through this".*
- Do not blame others, for example, colleagues.
- Be empathic and express concern where appropriate.
- Try not to be defensive or aggressive.
- Listen to the patient and explore their concerns.
- Agree an appropriate management plan, for example, raising the issue at the next practice meeting.
- Summarise the plan and ensure there are no other issues that have not been dealt with.
- Offer details of how the patient can make a formal complaint. A complaint to the practice manager will usually be acknowledged within two working days and responded to within ten working days, although this varies between practices.
- Housekeeping – it is also important to look after your own well-being.

Role play

Information for doctor	Additional information for role player
Patient: Mrs TT *Age*: 32 years *SH*: Lives with partner, unemployed, no children *PMH*: NIDDM *DH*: Metformin 500 mg TDS *Information*: You are a salaried GP.	*PC*: *"I've had a sore throat for over a week and I'm very angry because I've been trying to see a doctor for days and I have never been able to get an appointment".* *HPC*: Not happy with the appointment system. **No fever, earache, cough, rash, headache, neck stiffness or photophobia.** Has tried throat lozenges OTC and paracetamol but not working. *ICE*: **Wants antibiotics to get rid of the sore throat.** Will get angry if she doesn't get these unless a suitable explanation is given. *O/E*: Apyrexial; HR 70, regular; normal ENT and chest examination. Mild cervical lymphadenopathy.

Breaking bad news

- Breaking bad news is a duty which understandably many GPs dread, but is nevertheless a necessary skill to learn well.

Tips for breaking bad news

Preparation
- Arrange a face to face meeting and not a telephone consultation ideally.
- Ensure a private setting with no interruptions.
- Invite a relative or friend if appropriate.
- Prepare beforehand by familiarising yourself with the patient's clinical details.

Data gathering
- Discover what information the patient already knows or what they have been told so far – *"Before we start, do you mind me just asking what you understand about the tests and why they were done?"*.
- Discover what has happened since the patient was last seen – *"How have things been since you were last seen?"*.
- Give the patient a warning shot that difficult information is to follow, for example: *"I'm afraid that it looks more serious than we had hoped"* or *"I'm afraid that it is rather bad news"*.
- Share the information in small 'chunks', clearly and honestly, repeating the salient points. Allow pauses where appropriate.
- Avoid jargon.
- Continue to check the patient's understanding.
- Be aware of the patient's non-verbal cues as this can help to gauge the patient's need for further information.
- Show empathy, for example, *"I know that this must be very difficult for you"*.
- Address the patient's ideas, concerns and expectations.
- Enquire about the patient's social history – support network, occupation.

Clinical management
- Decide on a management plan which should include some sort of follow-up appointment and safety net.
- Offer some hope but this should also be tempered with realism.
- Offer a patient information leaflet if appropriate.
- Offer to make another appointment with spouse/relative or to speak to them on the phone.

Role play

Information for doctor	Additional information for role player
Patient: Mrs ZS	*PC:* "I was asked to come to get my biopsy results from the breast clinic". "Is there a problem?".
Age: 42 years	
SH: Married with 5 children	*HPC:* Felt a left breast lump 4 weeks ago. Has increased in size since. **Not painful. No nipple discharge. No skin tethering.** Otherwise feeling well.
PMH: Nil	
DH: Nil	
Information: Saw the salaried GP 4 weeks ago due to a breast lump. Was seen in the breast clinic 2 weeks ago and has come for her results. You are a locum GP.	*FH:* **No FH of breast cancer.**
	ICE: Worried it might be breast cancer.
Biopsy result: Adenocarcinoma of left breast.	

Patient with learning disabilities

- Learning disability is defined as a 'significantly reduced ability to understand new and complex information, to learn new skills (impaired intelligence), and with a reduced ability to cope independently (impaired social functioning)'. It starts before adulthood with a lasting effect on development. Often there are associated co-morbidities, for example, epilepsy, mental illness and behavioural disorders (*DoH White Paper*, 2001, *Valuing people: a new strategy for learning disabilities for the 21st century*).
- People with learning disabilities die 16 years younger than the general population (CIPOLD Report 2013).
- A consultation with a patient who has learning disabilities can be challenging for both the patient and the doctor.
- The patient may feel that their health needs have been neglected, whilst the doctor may feel frustrated by the potential difficulty in gathering the relevant clinical information to formulate a management plan.
- Evidence has shown that people with learning disabilities have much greater health needs than the general population, yet they don't access primary care as often as they need to (*NHS Primary Service Framework*, 2007, *Management of health for people with learning disabilities in primary care*).
- Management of patients with learning disabilities involves a multidisciplinary team approach.

Tips for data gathering and clinical management

- The people caring for the patient, whether the patient lives with their parents, or has a carer, or lives in a residential home, are all very useful sources of information.
- Listen to the patient and give them time to express their concerns.
- When history taking, ensure that the patient understands the questions asked and avoid using any jargon.
- It is important to try building a rapport with the patient, and ideally they should see the same GP each visit.
- When giving information, writing things down can be useful if the patient is literate. Drawing diagrams or giving patient information leaflets can also be helpful.
- All patients with learning disabilities should have at least an annual health check, and should have an individualised 'health action plan' (*DoH White Paper*, 2001, *Valuing people: a new strategy for learning disabilities for the 21st century*).
- A health check should include a minimum of:
  - provision of relevant health promotion advice
  - chronic illness and system enquiry
  - physical examination
  - consideration of whether the patient suffers from epilepsy, any mental health or behavioural problems

- specific syndrome check
- medication review
- review of co-ordination arrangements with other healthcare providers.
  - Always consider whether the patient is vulnerable or if there are any safeguarding issues.

Role play

Information for doctor	Additional information for role player
Patient: Mr TB *Age*: 36 years *SH*: Lives in a residential home for people with learning disabilities. *PMH*: Down syndrome, hypothyroidism, mild hearing impairment. *DH*: Levothyroxine 75 mcg OD *Information*: Was last seen by GP 8 months ago for ear infection. You are a salaried GP.	*PC*: *"I've got tummy pains doc", 'I've had it for a few days and it's really bad".* *HPC*: Lower abdominal pain, mainly left-sided. Intermittent pain. **Last opened bowels 5 days ago. No urinary symptoms. No D&V. No fever.** Not taken any painkillers so far. **Doesn't have much fibre in his diet. Doesn't drink much water.** *ICE*: Worried about his appendix. *O/E*: Apyrexial. HR 80, regular. BP 130/86. Abdo soft. Mild tenderness on left side of abdomen. No organomegaly. Palpable mass in LIF. Bowel sounds present.

Patient with hearing impairment

- Hearing impairment in general practice is a relatively common problem; however, research suggests that the needs of this patient group are poorly met in many GP surgeries (Patient UK, 2009, *Survey of people with mild to profound hearing loss*).
- The problems that patients with hearing impairment face include problems trying to book appointments, not hearing their name being called by the doctor, not being offered an interpreter, and not being able to understand the doctor.
- In the CSA exam there may be a hearing impaired patient, and they would most likely communicate by lip reading.
- When communicating with a hearing impaired patient, it is vital to ensure that you communicate clearly, with good face to face contact, and regularly check patient understanding.

Tips for dealing with hearing-impaired patients

- Always ask the patient at the beginning of the consultation how they wish to communicate.
- Always look at the patient when listening and speaking.
- Avoid looking at the patient's notes when talking to the patient – look at these before the patient enters.

- Ensure you are sitting in good light and keep your hands away from your face if the patient is lip reading.
- Speak clearly but not too slowly.
- Use hand gestures where appropriate.
- Don't exaggerate lip movements if the patient is lip reading.
- Keep a pen and paper handy in case you need to write anything down.
- Ask the patient to summarise what has been said to ensure understanding.
- Offer additional written material at the end of the consultation.
- Drawing diagrams to explain things may be especially useful in this case.

Role play

Information for doctor	Additional information for role player
Patient: Mrs RA *Age*: 48 years *SH*: Lives with husband and 3 children. Housewife *FH*: Nil *PMH*: IBS *DH*: Nil *Information*: You are a GP Registrar.	*PC*: *"I've been having problems with my hearing for the past month or so".* *HPC*: Can't hear on left side. **No tinnitus. No headache. No earache. No dizziness or vertigo.** Never had hearing tested before. **No trauma. No vomiting.** *ICE*: Worried she might be going deaf. **Would like a hearing test.** *O/E*: Decreased hearing on left side. Abnormal Weber's test – sound localised to right ear.

Patient refusing emergency management/hospital admission

- The GMC guidance states, "*You must respect a competent patient's decision to refuse an investigation or treatment, even if you think their decision is wrong or irrational.*"
- In these circumstances you can advise the patient of your clinical opinion, but you must not put pressure on them to accept your advice.
- GMC guidance states that in an emergency, "*you can provide treatment that is immediately necessary to save life or prevent deterioration in health without consent or, in exceptional circumstances, against the wishes of a person with parental responsibility*".

Assessment of patients refusing treatment

- Does the patient have capacity to make this decision? (see *Appendix 3*)
- Clearly explain your advice to the patient, e.g. "*My advice is that you need to go into hospital straight away for an alcohol detox programme*".
- Clarify the patient's understanding of the advice you have given.

- Ask them to repeat the information back to confirm understanding.
- Clearly explain the consequences of not following the advice you have given, e.g. *"If you don't go into hospital now there is a risk you may have another seizure which could be a risk to your life".*
- Try to show empathy and avoid sounding forceful.
- Even if the patient refuses admission or treatment, respect their wishes and offer an alternative form of management, if available.

Role play

Information for doctor	Additional information for role player
Patient: Mr RK *Age*: 68 years *PMH*: Type 2 diabetes, hypertension, MI 2008 *DH*: Metformin 1 g TDS, amlodipine 10 mg OD, ramipril 5 mg OD, aspirin 75 mg OD, atorvastatin 20 mg OD. *Information*: Mr K was given antibiotics for cellulitis 10 days ago by a locum GP and given a further course 5 days later. Cellulitis now spreading. You are a GP partner.	*PC*: *"I've been feeling feverish since last night". "The redness in my legs is now spreading up to my knee".* *HPC*: Nausea. No vomiting. **Painful leg**. *ICE*: Wants more antibiotic tablets. Definitely won't go into hospital as doesn't like hospitals. *O/E*: Temp 39°C. HR 110. Red hot leg to knee (spread from mid-calf previously). No tenderness at back of calf. Tender over shin.

Healthy people: promoting health and preventing disease

Hypercholesterolaemia

- Refers to a high level of lipids in the blood stream.
- It is more specifically defined as an elevation in total cholesterol, low density lipoproteins or triglycerides in the bloodstream.
- Fatty lumps called atheromas can develop in the lining of the blood vessels if the cholesterol remains high.
- A build up of atheroma can result in ischaemic heart disease, stroke, TIA or other arterial disease developing.
- Other risk factors for atheroma formation include high blood pressure, obesity, diabetes, unhealthy diet and strong family history.
- The figure below shows how you can illustrate the effect of atheromas on blood vessels.

Normal artery

Narrowing artery

Atheromas

Data gathering

Open questions

- *"I gather you recently had a cholesterol test done. Do you mind telling me what you understand about this test?"*
- *"What do you know about having high cholesterol?"*
- *"Tell me about your diet?"*

Focused/closed questions

HPC: *"Do you have any chest pain or shortness of breath?"* (red flags)

PMH: *"Do you have any history of high blood pressure, high cholesterol, heart disease or diabetes?"*

DH: Certain medications can raise cholesterol, e.g. antipsychotics, isotretinoin (roaccutane).

SH: Smoking/alcohol/illicit drug history? Exercise?

FH: *"Do any of your family have high cholesterol or heart disease?"*

ICE: *"Do you have any thoughts as to why your cholesterol is high?"*

Examination:
- blood pressure
- BMI
- cardiovascular system, including inspection for xanthelasma and tendon xanthomas.

Clinical management

Investigations
- Full lipid profile – total serum cholesterol, HDL, LDL, triglycerides.
- HbA1C.
- LFTs – if starting statins.
- Renal function and eGFR.
- TFTs – check TSH if dyslipidaemia is present.
- CK – check if symptomatic with unexplained muscle pain.

Explanation to patient
- Cholesterol is a fat made in the liver from the foods that we eat.
- A small amount of cholesterol is beneficial in keeping us healthy.
- If the cholesterol level is too high (approx. >5 mmol/l), there is an increased risk of developing heart problems or having a stroke.
- Cholesterol is carried in the bloodstream by particles called lipoproteins. There are two types of lipoproteins: low density lipoproteins (LDL) and high density lipoproteins (HDL). The LDL are often referred to as the 'bad' cholesterol as they are thought to be responsible for atheroma formation, whereas HDL are referred to as the 'good' cholesterol as they are thought to prevent atheroma formation.
- It is therefore important to keep the total cholesterol level down to an acceptable level (≤5 mmol/l), or for secondary prevention aim for total cholesterol <4 mmol/l.

Management
(based on *NICE* 2014 guideline CG181: *Cardiovascular disease: risk assessment and reduction, including lipid modification*)
- We should assess CV risk for primary prevention using the QRISK2 score (see guidelines for exceptions).
- Cardio-protective diet – fewer saturated fats, less alcohol, at least five portions of fruit and vegetables each day, and two portions of fish per week.
- Weight management and exercise – 30 minutes of at least moderate intensity exercise at least 5 days a week.
- Smoking cessation.

- Initiate statins for primary prevention of CVD if 10-year risk >10%. Atorvastatin 20 mg is the preferred choice for primary prevention. In secondary prevention patients should be offered a high dose of 80 mg atorvastatin. If statins are not tolerated other options include ezetimibe or fibrates.
- Lipids should be rechecked after 3 months and if a >40% reduction in non-HDL cholesterol has not been achieved, discuss adherence, optimize lifestyle advice and consider increasing the statin dose.
- Safety net – if on statins monitor LFTs within 3 months and then 12 monthly.

Role play

Information for doctor	Additional information for role player
Patient: Mrs HB *Age*: 46 years *PMH*: Hypertension *DH*: Ramipril 5 mg OD *Weight*: 96 kg (BMI 40) *Information*: Had a recent cholesterol test: total serum cholesterol 6.8 (NR: <5.2) serum LDL 4.2 (NR: 1.5–3.0); serum HDL 1.1 (NR: >1.0) serum triglycerides 2.0 (NR: <1.7) You are a locum GP.	*PC*: *"I have come to get my cholesterol results".* *HPC*: No symptoms. Feels well. **Cooks with a lot of oils and eats a lot of cheese. Also enjoys cakes. Inactive.** *SH*: **No alcohol intake. Non-smoker. Housewife.** *FH*: **Mother had high cholesterol. Father has diabetes.** *ICE*: Not keen to start a cholesterol tablet as doesn't like taking tablets. Would rather try to change her diet. Doesn't feel she has the time to exercise as busy looking after 3 children. *O/E*: BP 160/90. HR 75, regular. Heart sounds normal. Chest clear. No xanthelasma/tendon xanthomas.

Hypertension

- Blood pressure means the pressure of the blood in your arteries (blood vessels).
- Approximately half of all people over 65 years have high blood pressure (hypertension).
- It is recommended that GPs diagnose hypertension only after obtaining two or more elevated blood pressure readings on separate occasions.
- Risk factors for hypertension include obesity, inactivity, alcohol and smoking.
- Ambulatory blood pressure monitoring (ABPM) is recommended to confirm the diagnosis, defined as ABPM daytime mean of ≥135/85 (stage 1 hypertension).
- Home monitoring can be used as an alternative if ABPM is declined or not tolerated.
- Hypertension can result in an increased risk of ischaemic heart disease and stroke.

Data gathering

Open question

- *"Your recent blood pressure check has shown that your blood pressure is higher than normal. What do you understand about high blood pressure?"*

Focused/closed questions

HPC: *"Do you have any headaches or problems with your vision? Any chest pain?"*

PMH: *"Do you have any history of high blood pressure, high cholesterol, heart disease or stroke?"*

SH: Smoking/alcohol/illicit drug history? Diet? Exercise? Occupation? Stress?

FH: *"Does anyone else in the family have high blood pressure?"*

ICE: *"Do you have any thoughts as to why your blood pressure might be high?"*

Red flags:
- systolic BP >220 mmHg or diastolic BP >120 mmHg
- pregnant
- malignant hypertension – BP >180/110 mmHg with signs of papilloedema and/or retinal haemorrhage (refer same day to specialised care)

Examination:
- re-check BP
- fundoscopy
- BMI
- cardiovascular system

Clinical management

Investigations
- Bloods – U&Es, lipid profile and HbA1C.
- ECG.
- Urine dipstick – check for protein and blood (red flag if microscopic haematuria).
- Consider checking urinary catecholamines if young to rule out phaeochromocytoma.

Explanation to patient
- Blood pressure measurements consist of two readings – the top reading records the highest pressure in the arteries when the heart contracts. The bottom reading records the lowest pressure in the arteries as the heart relaxes between beats.
- If either of these readings are high then you have high blood pressure (above 140/90 mmHg).
- High blood pressure can be due to genetic factors, high salt or alcohol intake, lack of exercise or stress.
- If your blood pressure remains high you are at increased risk of having a heart attack or a stroke.
- It is therefore important that your blood pressure is kept within an acceptable range and it should be monitored regularly.

Management
(based on JBS3 Hypertension Guidance 2014)
- Lifestyle advice – low salt and high potassium diet, reduce alcohol intake, increase exercise, stop smoking.
- Offer anti-hypertensive medication to patients with a clinic BP >160/100, those with stage 2 hypertension or those with stage 1 hypertension and established CVD, CKD or evidence of target end organ damage.

BP: Start treatment if BP ↑ >180/110 → start on the day, if papilloedema/haemorrhage ↑ ref OTO.

ABPM ≥ 160/95 (stage 2 HTN) (or clinic consistently >160/100) ≥11

ABPM ≥ 135/85 (stage 1 HTN) → if co-morbidities ≥11

- In hypertensive patients aged 55 or older, or black patients of any age, the first choice drug for initial therapy is either a calcium channel blocker or a thiazide diuretic.
- In hypertensive patients younger than 55, the first choice is an ACE inhibitor (or angiotensin-II receptor antagonist if unable to tolerate an ACE inhibitor).
- Refer immediately if any signs of malignant hypertension (BP >180/110 mmHg with papilloedema +/− retinal haemorrhage) or phaeochromocytoma (signs include headache, palpitations and excessive sweating).
- Safety net – review hypertensive patients annually or more frequently if poorly controlled blood pressure. Advise patients to see GP or go to A&E if they develop any of the symptoms above.

Role play

Information for doctor	Additional information for role player
Patient: Mr JB *Age*: 57 years *SH*: Farm labourer, smokes 10 cigs/day, alcohol intake 30 units/wk *PMH*: Gout *DH*: Allopurinol 100 mg OD *Information*: Registered with practice last week. BP on registration 180/95 mmHg. You are a GP partner.	*PC*: *"I was asked to book an appointment to get my BP checked".* *HPC*: Feels well; no headache or visual symptoms. Doesn't understand why he needed to come back as he feels fine. **Eats a lot of takeaways. No exercise except for job.** *ICE*: No concerns. *O/E*: BP 175/98; weight 100 kg (BMI 34); CVS exam NAD.

Obesity

- Often classified as a BMI of over 30.
- BMI is defined as an individual's body weight (in kilograms) divided by the square of his or her height (in metres). It provides a good estimate as to whether an individual is in a healthy weight range by taking into consideration their height.
- In just less than 20 years obesity rates in the UK have doubled to 24% in men and 26% in women (*NICE*, 2014, *CG189: Obesity: identification, assessment and management*).
- It is important to assess the patient's motivation and readiness to change. A commonly used model includes the five stages of pre-contemplation, contemplation, preparation, action and maintenance.

Data gathering

Open questions
- *"Your current weight places you in the obese range... can you tell me a bit more about your lifestyle in terms of your diet and exercise levels?"*
- *"What do you think of your current weight?"*

Focused/closed questions

HPC: *"How much exercise do you do in an average week?"*

"Does your diet contain a lot of fatty &/or sugary foods?"

"Have you previously tried to lose weight?"

"What has prompted you to lose weight now?"

"Any breathlessness or chest pain?" (red flags)

"Any tiredness or problems sleeping?"

"Any bowel symptoms?"

Patient motivation/readiness to change:

"In the past month have you been actively trying to lose weight?"

"Are you seriously considering trying to lose weight to reach your goal in the next 6 months?"

"Have you maintained your desired weight for more than 6 months before?"

PMH: Any history of high blood pressure, high cholesterol or diabetes? Depression/stress? Eating disorder, e.g. binge eating?

SH: Smoking history? Alcohol? Occupation?

FH: *"Do any of your family have weight problems?"*

ICE: *"Do you have any particular concerns about your weight?"*

"What were you hoping we could do to help you?"

Examination:
- BMI (>25 overweight; >30 obese; >40 morbidly obese)
- BP
- cardiovascular system – to check for secondary problems

Clinical management

Investigations
- Blood test – lipid profile, HbA1C, U&Es, LFTs, TSH. LH/FSH in females if excluding PCOS.

Explanation to patient
- Obesity is defined as a BMI of over 30.
- The BMI provides a good estimate of how much of your body is made up of fat.
- When you are overweight or obese, it simply means that your energy intake exceeds energy expenditure.
- If you are overweight or obese you are at increased risk of developing health problems such as diabetes, high blood pressure, heart disease, or some types of cancer.

Management
- Low calorie/low fat diet (more fruit and vegetables, fish and lean meats, fewer sugary drinks, grilling instead of frying, etc.). Aim for 600 kcal/day deficit in combination with expert support and intensive follow-up for sustainable weight loss.
- Increase exercise – ideally 30 minutes exercise daily for 5 days a week. Consider exercise on prescription if available, and encourage patient to build activity into their day, e.g. climbing stairs at work instead of taking the lift.
- Decrease alcohol intake.

- Anti-obesity medications – Orlistat 120 mg TDS:
  - interferes with the way that fats are digested and absorbed in the body.
  - can only be prescribed for patients with a BMI of >30 or >28 with an associated health problem (*NICE*, 2014, *CG189: Obesity*).
  - side effects include fatty stools, excess wind and increased urgency.
  - patients must lose at least 5% of their body weight in the first 3 months to continue with this medication (*NICE*, 2014, *CG189: Obesity*).
- Bariatric surgery, e.g. gastric band/gastric bypass (NICE criteria for bariatric surgery includes BMI >40 or >35 with other co-morbidities such as type 2 diabetes, and when other treatments have failed (*NICE*, 2014, *CG189: Obesity*).
- Regular follow up providing ongoing support and encouragement.

Role play

Information for doctor	Additional information for role player
Patient: Mrs JN *Age*: 37 years *SH*: Married, works as chef. Non-smoker; 5 units alcohol/wk. *PMH*: NIDDM *DH*: Metformin 500 mg TDS *Information*: Had review with nurse last week: Weight 98 kg, BMI 38. You are a locum GP.	*PC*: "*I would like some of those weight loss tablets doctor*". *HPC*: Has been trying to lose weight for months. Feels that she eats healthily but still doesn't lose any weight. **Doesn't have time for exercise. Snacks at work. Typically skips breakfast. Eats chicken mayonnaise sandwich for lunch and often curry with rice for dinner.** *FH*: Nil. *ICE*: Would like some weight loss tablets. Wants to drop a few dress sizes but not keen on attending weight management programme as too busy with work. *O/E*: Weight 99 kg; BP 140/86; CVS exam – NAD.

Smoking cessation

- Cigarette smoking is the single greatest cause of illness and premature death in the UK.
- Approximately 100 000 people die each year in the UK as a result of smoking-related illnesses.
- Stopping smoking can be very beneficial to a person's health and well-being.
- Smoking cessation interventions should be individualised based on the patient history and readiness for change. Consider the five stage 'readiness for change' model below:
  - Pre-contemplation – *"I like to smoke"*
  - Contemplation – *"I like to smoke but I know I need to quit"*
  - Preparation – *"I'm ready to quit"*
  - Action – *"I'm no longer smoking but I still think about it from time to time"*
  - Maintenance – *"I used to smoke"*

Data gathering

Open questions
- *"So tell me a bit more about why you have decided to give up smoking?" "Why now?"*
- *"What are your thoughts and feelings about quitting smoking?"*

Focused/closed questions

HPC: *"How many cigarettes are you currently smoking a day?"*
"When did you first start smoking?"
"Have you ever tried to give up smoking before?" "What method did you use?"
"When is your predicted stop date?"
"When is your predicted stop date?"
"Any cough? Do you cough up any phlegm?"
"Any breathlessness, coughing up blood or weight loss?" (red flags)

PMH: Any medical conditions?

DH: Do you take any regular medications? (bupropion taken with certain medications, e.g. anti-psychotics or anti-depressants, increases the risk of seizures)

FH: *"Is there any history of cancer, lung disease or heart disease in the family?"*

SH: Alcohol/illicit drug history? Who lives with you at home? Support? Occupation?

ICE: *"What help were you hoping for in terms of stopping smoking?"*
"What do you understand about the different ways to stop smoking?

Examination: Nothing specific although if there are signs of chest symptoms do a respiratory examination.

Clinical management

Investigations
- Nothing specific although if there are any chest symptoms consider spirometry or CXR.

Explanation to patient
- Nicotine is a drug that is inhaled from the tobacco in cigarettes.
- Nicotine is the addictive ingredient in cigarettes – as the blood level of nicotine falls, people develop withdrawal symptoms, for example, anxiety, irritability, headaches and difficulty concentrating.
- By replacing the nicotine or mimicking the effects of the nicotine, there are substitution treatments that can help when trying to stop smoking.

Management
- Patient information leaflet – www.patient.co.uk - '*Tips to help you stop smoking*'.
- Local NHS smoking cessation service or support groups.
- Self help, telephone support or one-to-one counselling.

- Nicotine replacement therapy – stops or reduces the symptoms of nicotine withdrawal (available in gum, patches, lozenges, etc.).
- Varenicline (Champix) – mimics the effects of nicotine on the body. Standard treatment course is 12 weeks. Side effects include nausea, insomnia, abnormal dreams and less commonly mood changes. Should not be used if under 18, pregnant, breast-feeding or if severe renal disease. Use with caution in patients with a history of psychiatric illness.
- Buproprion (Zyban) – alters the level of some chemicals in the brain that seem to relieve the withdrawal symptoms associated with stopping smoking. Standard treatment course is 8 weeks. Side effects include dry mouth, insomnia and, rarely, seizures. It should not be used if under 18, pregnant, breast-feeding or if the patient has ever had epilepsy or a seizure. Also not advisable in certain psychiatric conditions. See BNF for further details.
- E-cigarettes – these are electrical devices that mimic cigarette smoking and often contain nicotine. They may be safer than normal cigarettes but we do not yet know the long-term effects of the vapour on the body. Recent study findings show that e-cigarettes can be effective in helping people to quit smoking.
- Offer regular follow-up and support.

Role play

Information for doctor	Additional information for role player
Patient: Mrs JS *Age*: 42 years *SH*: Receptionist, married, lives with husband and 2 children. *PMH*: Myocardial infarction 2011 *DH*: Aspirin 75 mg OD; simvastatin 40 mg nocte. *Information*: You are a GP Registrar	*PC*: *"I would like to give up smoking".* *HPC*: Has smoked 20 cigs/day for past 25 years. Has not tried to quit before. Her children have been nagging her to quit. No shortness of breath and no weight loss. **No cough or haemoptysis.** *SH*: Alcohol 12 units/wk *ICE*: **Keen to quit smoking as had a heart attack last year which scared her. Would like to try Zyban as a friend recommended it.**

Dietary advice for malnourished patients

- Malnutrition is a state in which a deficiency of nutrients such as energy, protein, vitamins and minerals results in measurable adverse effects on body composition, function and clinical outcome (*NICE*, 2012, *CG32: Nutrition support in adults*).
- According to NHS Choices, around one in three people admitted to hospital or care homes in the UK are found to be malnourished or at risk of malnourishment.
- It is defined as:
  - BMI <18.5
  - Unintentional weight loss of >10% within the past 3–6 months
  - BMI <20, and unintentional weight loss of >5% within the past 3–6 months

- NICE states we should 'screen' vulnerable patients, and when you have clinical concern that they may have malnutrition, use a validated tool such as the MUST tool (www.bapen.org.uk).

Data gathering

Open questions
- *"What is your appetite like?"*
- *"Can you take me through a typical day's food and drink?"*

Focused/closed questions

HPC: *"Have you noticed any recent weight loss?"*
"Have you been eating less recently?"
"Have you been unwell recently?"
"Have you had any nausea or vomiting?"
"Have you had any diarrhoea?"
"Have you had any difficulty swallowing?"
"Are your clothes tighter or looser than usual?"

PMH: *"Have you had any previous problems with poor diet or weight loss?"*

DH: Certain medications can cause weight loss, e.g. levothyroxine, methylphenidate. Check compliance with medications, especially if self-neglect

SH: Living and cooking arrangements? Any help with cooking? Do you live alone? Any friends/relatives who can help if required?

ICE: *"Are you concerned about your dietary habits and your weight?"*

Examination:
- BMI.
- General appearance – cachectic, skin pallor, sunken eyes,
- Hair – thin, easily plucked.
- Mouth – tongue fissuring.

Clinical management

Investigations
- 'MUST' calculator.
- FBC, U&Es, LFTs, TFTs, magnesium, ferritin, folate, B12, zinc, glucose, coeliac serology.

Explanation to patient
- You are malnourished, which means your diet does not contain the right amount of nutrients or you are not absorbing them properly.
- Malnutrition makes you more vulnerable to catching infections. It also delays wound healing and reduces the function of your heart and lungs. It can be potentially fatal if not treated.
- If you are undernourished, you may need to increase the nutritional content of your food, with or without taking nutritional supplements.
- The best way to prevent malnutrition is to have a healthy, balanced diet.

Management

(based on *NICE*, 2012, *CG32: Nutrition support for adults* and *RCGP Malnutrition Pathway*)

- Ideally refer to a community dietitian/specialist nutrition nurse; set goals and monitor progress.
- 'Food first' approach at all times to maximise oral intake.
- Advise high calorie/high protein foods, e.g. cheese, butter, cream, full fat milk, etc.
- Small frequent meals and snacks.
- Advise fortifying diets and nutritional 'calorie boosters', e.g. peanut butter, mayonnaise, honey, cashew nuts, coconut cream.
- Consider adding a multivitamin and mineral supplement.
- Prescribe additional oral nutritional supplements in those at high risk, or who have eaten little or nothing for 5 days, or have poor absorption due to illness:
  - prescribe 1–3 oral nutritional supplements per day to be used in addition to the above dietary advice
  - assess after 4–6 weeks to monitor use and compliance
  - if long-term need, continue 2 oral nutritional supplements per day and monitor every 12 weeks.

Role play

Information for doctor	Additional information for role player
Patient: Mrs PS *Age:* 86 *PMH:* Hypertension, osteoporosis *DH:* Amlodipine 10 mg OD. Alendronic acid 70 mg once weekly, calcichew D3 forte OD. *Information:* You are a GP partner. Patient's husband died 8 months ago and she has struggled on her own since then.	*PC:* "I am feeling cold and tired all the time". *HPC:* **Constipated. Not eating well. Poor appetite.** Weight loss – 6 kg over past 6–8 months. *SH:* Lives alone. No carers. Poor family support. *ICE:* Hoping for a blood test and also some extra support at home. *O/E:* BMI 17. Cachectic. Thin hair. BP 90/60.

Genetics in primary care

Antenatal screening for Down syndrome

- Down syndrome is a chromosomal abnormality in which there is an extra copy of chromosome number 21 (often known as trisomy 21).
- Characteristic features of Down syndrome include macroglossia, epicanthic folds, upslanting palpebral fissures and a single transverse palmar crease. Individuals with Down syndrome have a higher incidence of congenital heart defects, gastro-oesophageal reflux, recurrent ear infections and thyroid problems.
- Down syndrome can be diagnosed either before birth (antenatally) or after birth.
- The latest NICE guidelines recommend that all pregnant women should be offered screening for Down syndrome.
- There are two different types of tests that can be done in pregnancy – a screening test and a diagnostic test.
  - Screening test – looks at the chance of a baby being born with Down syndrome in the current pregnancy.
  - Diagnostic test – amniocentesis or chorionic villus sampling is used to give a definite diagnosis as to whether or not the fetus has Down syndrome. Usually only done if the screening test indicates a high chance of Down syndrome (usually >1/250 risk).
- Screening tests used include:
  - The combined test is the one which NICE currently recommends. This includes a nuchal translucency scan (measures the size of the nuchal pad at the nape of the fetal neck) and blood tests for serum PAPP-A and β-hCG (undertaken between 11 weeks and 13 weeks[+6]).
  - Amniocentesis – a sample of amniotic fluid is taken from the amniotic sac using a fine needle. This is normally done at 15 weeks of gestation and carries an additional 1% risk of miscarriage.
  - CVS – a small sample of tissue is taken from part of the placenta called the chorionic villi. Normally done at 11[+0]–13[+6] weeks of gestation (*RCOG*, 2010: *Green-top guideline 8: Amniocentesis and chorionic villus sampling*) and carries an approximately 2% risk of miscarriage.

Data gathering

Open question

- *"What do you know about Down syndrome and the antenatal screening tests available?".*

Focused/closed questions

HPC: *"Is this your first pregnancy?"*

If not, any problems in previous pregnancies? Miscarriages? TOP?

"Have you had Down's screening in previous pregnancies? Any concerns?"

SH: "Who lives with you at home?" Occupation? Support?

FH: Does anyone in the family have Down syndrome?

ICE: *"Do you have concerns about the risk of Down syndrome?"*

"Do you know anyone with Down syndrome?"

Examination:
- BP
- Routine antenatal examination

Clinical management

Investigations

- Screening tests (see www.patient.co.uk article *'Prenatal Screening and Diagnosis of Down's Syndrome'* for further details).
- Amniocentesis.
- CVS.

Explanation to patient

- Down syndrome is a genetic disorder where a person inherits an extra copy of one chromosome. The additional genetic material changes the finely tuned balance of the body, resulting in characteristic physical features and affects the normal physical development.

Management

- Give patient information leaflet.
- Follow up after the screening/diagnostic tests.
- Refer to obstetrician and geneticist if Down syndrome confirmed antenatally.

Role play

Information for doctor	Additional information for role player
Patient: Mrs TW *Age*: 40 years *PMH*: Hypothyroidism *DH*: Levothyroxine 100 mcg daily *SH*: Lives with husband, works as a solicitor, currently 8 weeks pregnant (1st pregnancy) *Information*: You are a salaried GP.	PC: Would like referral for antenatal Down syndrome screening and would like to know more about what the screening entails. HPC: Has heard about amniocentesis but was told there were some other tests available. LMP 8 weeks ago. No vaginal bleeding and no abdominal pain. Feels well otherwise. ICE: **Worried about the risk of Down syndrome due to her age. Her sister has a child with Down syndrome.** Would like the GP to explain the different options available.

Screening for sickle cell disease

- Antenatal screening for sickle cell diseases and thalassaemias should now be offered routinely to all women as early as possible in pregnancy, ideally by 10 weeks (NICE update: *NICE, 2008; CG62: Antenatal care*).
- Sickle cell disease is most common in people of African–Caribbean descent.
- Sickle cell disease affects the normal oxygen-carrying capacity of red blood cells due to a change in the biochemistry of haemoglobin. When deoxygenated red blood cells are unable to pass freely through capillaries, they form clusters instead and these block blood vessels. This blockage prevents oxygenation of the tissues in the affected areas, resulting in tissue hypoxia and consequent intense pain (known as sickle cell crisis). The other symptoms of sickle cell disease include severe anaemia, damage to major organs and infections. There is also an increased risk of stroke. Average life expectancy is about 50 years.
- For a baby to be affected with sickle cell disease both parents must have the sickle cell gene.
- Sickle cell trait occurs in people with one sickle cell gene and one normal gene. People with sickle cell trait do not usually have any clinical manifestation of illness.
- Pregnant women and couples planning to conceive may want to know whether they have sickle cell trait, because if they both have the gene their child might inherit sickle cell disease.

Data gathering

Open question
- *"What do you know about sickle cell conditions and the antenatal screening available?"*

Focused/closed questions
HPC: *"Is this your first pregnancy?"*
If not, any previous problems, for example miscarriages, TOP?
"Have you or your partner ever been screened for sickle cell trait before?"
"Have you or your partner ever had problems with recurrent infections or lethargy before?"

FH: *"Do you know of any family history of sickle cell disease or trait?"*

DH Do you take any regular medications?

SH: Smoking/alcohol/illicit drug history? Who lives with you at home? Support? Occupation?

ICE: *"Do you have any worries/concerns about sickle cell screening?"*
"Do you know anyone with sickle cell disease?"

Clinical management

Investigations
- Blood test called haemoglobin electrophoresis (offer to father also if mother carries the sickle cell gene).
- FBC – check Hb.

Explanation to patient
- Sickle cell disease is an inherited blood disorder which causes the red cells in the bloodstream to become sickle-shaped.
- When sickle-shaped cells block small blood vessels, less blood can reach that part of the body. This can result in damage to those affected tissues. This is what causes the complications of sickle cell disease.

Management
- Pre- and post-test counselling.
- Give information leaflet on sickle cell screening (http://sct.screening.nhs.uk/index.php).
- Refer to obstetrician and haematologist if both parents are carriers of the sickle cell gene.

Role play

Information for doctor	Additional information for role player
Patient: Ms CC *Age*: 28 years *SH*: Retail assistant. *DH*: Nil *Information*: Saw locum GP 1 week ago for antenatal booking – 6 weeks pregnant. White British ethnic origin.	*PC*: "I would like to get screened for the sickle cell gene as my partner has sickle cell trait and I'm currently pregnant." *HPC*: Never been screened before. **Doesn't know much about sickle cell disease.** No symptoms. Has had nausea but no other pregnancy related problems so far. *ICE*: Would like to find out more about screening and sickle cell disease. First pregnancy.

Cystic fibrosis

- Autosomal recessive condition mainly affecting the lungs, pancreas and digestive system.
- Symptoms begin in early childhood and include recurrent chest infections, malabsorption of food and failure to thrive.
- Treatment includes antibiotics, pancreatic enzyme replacements, chest physiotherapy and mucolytics.
- Approximately 1 in 25 people of Caucasian descent are carriers of the cystic fibrosis gene in the UK.

Data gathering

Open question
- *"Please can you tell me a bit more about your concerns?"*

Focused/closed questions

HPC: *"Have you been pregnant before? If so, any miscarriages or termination of pregnancies?"*
"Have you had any problems with antenatal scans before?"
"Have you or your partner been tested for the CF gene before?"
"Do you have children with any symptoms such as poor weight gain or recurrent chest infections?"

FH: *"Does anyone in the family have cystic fibrosis?"*

ICE: *"What concerns do you have about the possibility of your child/baby having cystic fibrosis?"*
"Do you know anyone with cystic fibrosis?"

Examination: Routine antenatal examination (if patient is pregnant)

Clinical management

Investigations
- Genetic testing prenatally – blood test or scrapings from the inside of the mouth can be used to check for the cystic fibrosis gene in the parents.
- Antenatal testing – uses chorionic villus sampling and is carried out from 10 weeks of pregnancy (only offered to mothers who are thought to be at high risk of having a child with the disease). Amniocentesis can also be performed between 15 and 20 weeks of pregnancy.
- After birth, a sweat test can be used to diagnose cystic fibrosis and blood from the Guthrie heel prick test is routinely screened for cystic fibrosis by checking for increased levels of immuno-reactive trypsinogen (IRT) at around 7 days of age.

Explanation to patient
- In order to get cystic fibrosis you have to inherit two cystic fibrosis genes, one from your mother and one from your father.
- In cystic fibrosis, a pair of genes on chromosome 7 don't work properly.
- These genes are responsible for the way cells handle salt and water and they control mucus secretions. When you have cystic fibrosis water and salt aren't transported out of cells so efficiently and as a result, the mucus secretions are thicker than normal; these sticky secretions are difficult to clear from the body leading to increased lung infections and damage to the digestive system.

Management
- If one or both parents carry the cystic fibrosis gene, refer for genetic counselling.
- Provide a patient information leaflet.
- If cystic fibrosis is confirmed, management requires a multidisciplinary team approach including specialist nurses, physiotherapists and dietitians.

- Treatments include physiotherapy, antibiotics, inhalers and nebulisers for respiratory symptoms, and enzyme supplements and high fat/carbohydrate diet for digestive problems.
- Patients with cystic fibrosis should have an annual flu and pneumococcal vaccine.
- In severe cases a heart/lung transplant may be necessary.

Role play

Information for doctor	Additional information for role player
Patient: Mrs JT *Age*: 31 years *SH*: Married, has 1 child with cystic fibrosis *PMH*: Asthma *DH*: Salbutamol 1–2 puffs PRN, beclomethasone 1 puff BD. *Information*: You are a GP Partner.	*PC*: Currently pregnant and worried about the risk of cystic fibrosis. *HPC*: Would like to get checked for whether the 2nd child will have cystic fibrosis. 8 weeks pregnant with same partner. Current child 3 years old and has spent a lot of time in hospital with respiratory symptoms. *ICE*: Very worried about the 2nd child also having CF. Wants further screening. Patient not sure she would want to continue with the pregnancy if CF is confirmed.

Care of acutely ill people

Suicidal patient

- Suicide can be described as a fatal act of self harm, initiated with the intention of ending one's own life.
- It is recognised as one of the most urgent public health concerns of our time (*BMJ*, 2015; 350: h783).
- Self harm describes the deliberate act of harming oneself.
- All health professionals should be vigilant of patients who express a desire to harm themselves, and these patients should have a suicide risk assessment undertaken.
- Risk factors for suicide include male gender, elderly, unemployed, history of mental illness or past suicide attempt, alcohol or drug abuse and poor social support.

Data gathering

Open questions
- *"Please can you tell me how you are currently feeling, and what has triggered these suicidal thoughts?"*
- *"How do you feel about the future?"*

Focused/closed questions

HPC:	*"How is your sleep/your concentration/your energy levels/your mood/your self-esteem?"*
	"Have you had thoughts of ending it all?"
	"Have you made specific plans for suicide? If so, what are these plans?"
	See suicide risk assessment below for further questions.
PMH:	Any past history of psychiatric illness? Any previous history of suicide/self harm?
DH:	*"Are you on any regular medications such as anti-depressants?"*
SH:	*"Is there anyone with you at home who can offer you support?"*
	Smoking history/alcohol/illicit drug use? Occupation? Farmers and healthcare practitioners are at higher risk.
FH:	Any FH of suicide/mental illness?
Examination:	Mental state examination (see *Appendix 3*).

Clinical management

Investigations

- Suicide risk assessment
  - *"Do you have any plan to harm yourself or others?"* (red flag)
  - *"Have you been thinking about this for a while or are these just fleeting thoughts?"*
  - *"How do you plan to end your life?"*
  - *"How seriously do you intend on acting on these thoughts?"* (red flag)
  - *"What would stop you?"*
  - *"Any previous suicide attempts or self harming episodes – how many?"* (red flag)
  - *"Any history of substance abuse?"*
  - *"Have you ever been in trouble with the police before?" "Have you ever been in prison before?"*
  - *"Any current contributing life stressors (financial, relationships, family, etc)?"*
  - *"Any symptoms of depression or psychosis?"*
  - *"Do you have any hope for the future?"*
  - *"Do you have any chronic medical conditions/terminal illness that may be contributing?"*
  - *"Do you feel isolated, lonely, angry or impulsive?"*
  - *"How do you cope with these issues?" "Do you feel able to talk to anyone about your problems?"*

Management

- If low suicide risk, offer regular follow-up and consider referral to the local mental health services.
- If moderate–high suicide risk refer urgently to the mental health crisis team.
- Give contact details of the Samaritans or the local crisis team if appropriate, and formulate an action plan to help resist suicidal thoughts.
- Always safety net – inform them of how they can access help if things get worse.

Role play

Information for doctor	Additional information for role player
Patient: Mr JS *Age:* 23 years *SH:* Lives alone, unemployed. Previous IVDU – on methadone. 30 units alcohol weekly. Smokes 20 cigarettes daily. *PMH:* Depression, previous psychiatric admission due to severe depression 2009. No forensic history. *DH:* Mirtazepine 60 mg. Methadone 60 mg OD. *Information:* You are a locum GP.	*PC:* *"I can't carry on like this" "I don't feel like living any more".* *HPC:* No specific plans for suicide. Feels hopeless as no job and struggling to pay bills. Low mood: **Doesn't feel able to talk to family. Waking up several times in the night. Poor concentration.** No previous suicide or self harm attempts. Feels little hope for the future. **No plan to harm others. His family would be what would stop him from suicide.** *ICE:* **Would like some urgent help as feels suicidal.**

Chest pain

- Can be divided into cardiac, respiratory, musculoskeletal or gastrointestinal causes.
- It is important to exclude a life threatening cause of chest pain, such as a myocardial infarction or a pulmonary embolism.

Data gathering

Open question
- *"Please can you describe the chest pain that you've been experiencing?"*

Focused/closed questions
HPC: *"Where is the site of the chest pain? Does the pain spread anywhere else?"*
"What type of pain is it?"
"Is the pain intermittent or constant?"
"How long has the pain lasted for?"
"How severe is the pain out of 10?"
"Is the pain present at rest or only on exertion?"
"Does anything make the pain better/worse?"
"Have you coughed up any blood or noticed any calf pain?" (red flags)
Any SOB, palpitations, cough or vomiting?
Any sweating or clamminess? (red flag)
"Any recent long haul flights or periods of immobility?"
PMH: Any previous heart attack or angina? Any previous surgery?
DH: *"Are you on any regular medications?"*
SH: Smoking/alcohol/illicit drug history? Occupation?
ICE: *"Do you have any idea what might be causing this chest pain?"*
"Are you concerned about anything in particular?"
"How has this pain been affecting you?"
Examination:
- BP, pulse, temperature and pulse oximetry
- Cardiac and respiratory examination
- Examine chest wall for any tenderness
- Examine calves for any swelling (DVT)
- Abdominal examination if indicated from the history

Clinical management

Investigations
- Routine bloods – FBC, U&Es, LFTs, TFTs, CRP/plasma viscosity, HbA1C, cardiac enzymes and lipids
- ECG
- CXR – if indicated

Management
- Depends on the diagnosis:
  - For non-acute chest pain consider referral to the rapid access chest pain clinic (NICE recommends same day referral if suspected ACS symptoms within the last 72 hours but no current chest pain).
  - If acute chest pain or any suggestion of a pulmonary embolus, refer urgently to A&E by ambulance (give GTN spray and 300 mg aspirin immediately).
- Safety net – if pain not improving or if worsening to return to GP or go straight to A&E.

Role play

Information for doctor	Additional information for role player
Patient: Mr JC *Age*: 53 years *SH*: Lives with wife and 2 children. Estate agent. *PMH*: Hypertension *DH*: Amlodipine 5 mg OD. *Information*: Saw nurse 1 week ago for BP check (150/89 mmHg). You are a GP Registrar.	*PC*: Chest pain. *HPC*: Pain in centre of chest which started yesterday. No radiation. Intermittent pain on exertion only. Slight SOB. No palpitations or cough. No fever and no sweating. No calf pain. No recent immobility. *FH*: Father had MI aged 60 years. *ICE*: Worried about his heart. Hoping for a scan to check his heart. *O/E*: Cardiac and respiratory examination – NAD. No chest wall or calf tenderness. BP 160/90.

Meningitis

- Inflammation of the meningeal coverings of the brain
- Most commonly caused by a bacterial or viral infection
- If bacteria multiply and release toxins into the blood, it can cause septicaemia which is life-threatening. Collectively, both meningitis and septicaemia are referred to as meningococcal disease.
- There are approximately 600–700 new cases per year in the UK, most of which occur in children under 5
- In the UK from September 2015, babies born on or after 1 July 2015 are being offered a meningitis B vaccine available on the NHS. It is recommended for babies aged 8 weeks, followed by a second dose at 16 weeks and a booster at one year

Data gathering

Open question
- *"What concerns do you have about your child?"*

Focused/closed questions

HPC: *"Have you noticed a rash on your child?"*

"Any fever, neck stiffness, headache, vomiting or sensitivity to light?" (red flags)

"Has your child been more drowsy or floppy than usual?" (red flags)

"Has your child been more irritable or crying more than usual?"

"Has your child been feeding OK?"

"Has your child had any episodes of fitting?" (red flags)

"Have you noticed any changes with his/her breathing?"

"Has your child been passing urine as usual?" (red flag if decreased urine output)

"Do you have any concerns about your child's growth and development?"

PMH: Any previous history of infections or illnesses?

SH: Where are you currently living? University/school accommodation?

FH: Any family history of any illnesses?

ICE: *"What do you think might be causing his/her symptoms?"*

Examination:
- Check temperature, RR, HR, BP, O_2 sats, neurological condition, CRT.
- Parents can check temperature and do the 'glass test' if at home.

Clinical management

Investigations
- If meningitis is suspected, refer directly to hospital immediately (**no need for any investigations in primary care**).
- Blood tests – FBC, U&Es, CRP, blood glucose.
- Urine MC&S.

Explanation to patient
- Meningitis is a swelling of the tissues around the brain and is usually caused by an infection.
- The symptoms often develop quickly and urgent treatment is needed with antibiotic injections. An antibiotic injection would be given immediately by the GP if suspected bacterial meningitis or meningococcal septicaemia. The patient would also be transferred to secondary care as an emergency by dialling 999.
- If meningitis is suspected, when in hospital a sample of fluid will most likely be taken from around the spinal cord to determine the cause.

Management
- Prevention – children are now routinely immunised against meningococcal group C and also *Haemophilus influenza* B. Immunisation against meningitis B started in September 2015.
- If bacterial meningitis is suspected in the community, immediately call 999. Give IM benzylpenicillin (300 mg if under 1 yr, 600 mg if 1–9 years, 1200 mg if 10 years plus) but do not delay transfer to hospital in order to give this. Give prophylaxis to close contacts.
- Notify the HPA on 'suspicion' of meningitis or meningococcal sepsis.

- Safety net – if there is a low risk of meningococcal disease the patient can be observed at home, but should be advised to go straight to A&E if they become more unwell or develop any signs of meningitis. Also arrange to review the following day in the GP surgery.

Role play

Information for doctor	Additional information for role player
Patient: Mr TD *Age*: 18 years *SH*: College student, non-smoker *PMH*: Nil *DH*: Nil *FH*: Nil *Information*: Called the practice this morning for an emergency appointment due to headache and fever. You are a salaried GP.	*PC*: Woke up this morning with fever, severe headache and rash. *HPC*: Generalised headache, photophobia and rash on his trunk. **Also loss of appetite. Very lethargic today. No vomiting. Slight neck discomfort.** *ICE*: **Mum worried about meningitis as someone in his college recently had this, and TD didn't have his meningitis immunisation.** *O/E*: Temp. 38.9°C, photophobia, neck stiffness, petechial non-blanching rash on the chest. Kernig's and Brudzinski's signs positive.

Head injury

- Minor head injuries and knocks to the head are common, especially in children.
- It is unusual for there to be any damage to the brain if there is no loss of consciousness and no severe head trauma.
- Occasionally, a head injury can cause damage to the blood vessels which may leak into the brain or into the area between the brain and skull (subdural haemorrhage). Although rare, this is potentially very serious because it can cause pressure to build up in the brain.
- Symptoms of bleeding or damage to the brain may not develop immediately, and in some cases may take several hours, days or even weeks.
- Red flag symptoms include loss of consciousness, vomiting, drowsiness, fitting and worsening headache. Always consider non-accidental injury especially in younger children.

Data gathering

Open question

- *"Please can you tell me a bit more about the head injury."*

Focused/closed questions

HPC: *"How did the head injury happen?"*
"When did it happen?"
"What was the mechanism of the injury?"
"Were you wearing any head protection?"

"Since the injury have you suffered with a headache? If so, is it worsening?" (red flag)
"Any vomiting?" (red flag)
"Any loss of consciousness?" (red flag)
"Have you been feeling more sleepy/drowsy since the head injury?" (red flag)

PMH: Any bleeding disorders? Any previous head injuries?

DH: *"Do you take any regular medications?"* (specifically enquire about aspirin, warfarin, etc.)

SH: Alcohol/drug history?

ICE: *"What concerns do you have about the head injury?"*

Examination:
- Neurological examination – including GCS.
- Assess for signs of a basal skull fracture – look for bruising around eyes (panda eyes) or ears (Battle's sign) and CSF/blood coming from ears and/or nose.

Clinical management

(based on *NICE*, 2014, *CG176: Head injury* and *SIGN*, 2009, *Guideline 110: Early management of patients with a head injury*)

Investigations
- CT head – only if red flags and after referring urgently to secondary care.

Management
- Analgesia – paracetamol, ibuprofen (avoid opiates if possible).
- Provide information leaflet with advice on what symptoms to look out for and when to seek further medical help.
- Refer to A&E if any red flags.
- SIGN guidelines: adult patients with any of the following signs or symptoms should be referred to hospital for further investigation:
  - GCS <15 at initial assessment
  - post-traumatic seizure
  - focal neurological signs
  - signs of a skull fracture
  - loss of consciousness
  - severe and persistent headache
  - repeated vomiting (two or more occasions)
  - post-traumatic amnesia >5 mins
  - retrograde amnesia >30 mins
  - high risk mechanism of injury
  - any history of bleeding/clotting disorder or current anticoagulation therapy
  - current alcohol or drug intoxication

In addition to the above referral criteria, children with head injuries should be referred if:

- clinical suspicion of non-accidental injury
- significant medical co-morbidity (e.g. learning difficulties, autism)
- difficulty making a full assessment
- not accompanied by a responsible adult or unsuitable social circumstances.

General head injury advice

- If possible, avoid staying at home alone for the first 48 hours after a head injury.
- Show a relative or friend the head injury advice leaflet so they too know what symptoms to look out for.
- Avoid any alcohol, drugs and ideally sleeping tablets for the following few days.
- It is often advised that you should not play contact sports for three weeks following a head injury.
- Do not drive or operate machinery until you feel completely recovered.

Role play

Information for doctor	Additional information for role player
Patient: Mr KM *Age*: 46 years *SH*: Lives with wife and 20 year old son. Lorry driver. *PMH*: Hypertension *DH*: Amlodipine 5 mg OD *FH*: Nil *Information*: You are a GP registrar. Not a frequent attender. Patient has booked an appointment to discuss a head injury.	*PC*: *"I hit my head at work yesterday and just thought I should get it checked out"* *HPC*: Hit head on forks of forklift truck at work. Cut head and has had headache since. **Not worsening. No vomiting. No LOC. No drowsiness.** Wasn't wearing helmet. *SH*: Alcohol intake 30 units weekly. Non-smoker. *ICE*: **Wife worried due to headache.** Took day off work today and wife has been with him. *O/E*: GCS 15/15. BP 140/80. Neuro exam – NAD.

Ectopic pregnancy

- An ectopic pregnancy can present with a variety of symptoms, most commonly abdominal or pelvic pain, amenorrhoea, missed period, or vaginal bleeding.
- Other less common symptoms, which may still be significant, include gastrointestinal symptoms, dizziness, shoulder tip pain, urinary symptoms, pain on defecation or passage of tissue.
- 12% of ectopic pregnancies are missed at initial presentation.
- Consider in any women of child-bearing age presenting with lower abdominal/pelvic pain with or without PV bleeding.

Data gathering

Open question

- *"Please can you tell me about the pain you are experiencing?"*

Focused/closed questions

HPC: *"When did the bleeding start?"*

"How much are you bleeding? Colour? Consistency?"

"Where is the tummy pain? What type of pain is it? Does it spread anywhere? When did it start? Is it constant?"

"When was your last period?"

"Are you sexually active at the moment?"

"Have you been using contraception?"

PMH: Have you had any similar problems in the past? Any previous operations of the abdomen or pelvis?

FH: Any family history of any problems relating to the abdomen or pelvis?

SH: Who lives with you? Are they supportive? Alcohol/drug history?

ICE: *"Is there anything in particular you are concerned about?"*

Examination:
- BP, pulse.
- Abdominal examination.
- If no abdominal pain/tenderness perform pelvic examination. (Do not test for adnexal tenderness as this risks rupturing the ectopic if present).

Clinical management

(*NICE*, 2012, *CG154: Ectopic pregnancy and miscarriage*)

Investigations
- Pregnancy test.
- Ultrasound scan – arranged via the early pregnancy assessment unit (EPAU).

Explanation to patient
- An ectopic pregnancy is when a fertilised egg implants itself outside of the womb, usually in one of the Fallopian tubes.
- This means the egg will not develop into a baby.
- Occasionally an ectopic pregnancy doesn't cause any noticeable symptoms; however, most women have symptoms that become apparent between weeks 5 and 14 of pregnancy.

Management
- Refer women who are haemodynamically unstable, or in whom there is significant concern about the degree of pain or bleeding, directly to A&E.
- Refer immediately to an EPAU service (or out-of-hours gynaecology service) women with a positive pregnancy test and the following on examination:
  ○ pain and abdominal tenderness *or*
  ○ pelvic tenderness *or*
  ○ cervical motion tenderness.
- Refer to an EPAU service (or out-of-hours gynaecology service) women with bleeding or other symptoms and signs of early pregnancy complications who have:

- o pain *or*
- o a pregnancy of 6 weeks' gestation or more *or*
- o a pregnancy of uncertain gestation. The urgency of this referral depends on the clinical situation.
- In pregnancies of less than 6 weeks' gestation and bleeding with no pain:
  - o refer to EPAU if bleeding continues after 6 weeks' pregnancy or if symptoms of an ectopic pregnancy develop
  - o if bleeding settles, repeat pregnancy test after 7 days to determine if they have had a miscarriage.

Role play

Information for doctor	Additional information for role player
Patient: Miss RK *Age*: 26 years *PMH*: Nil. No previous pregnancies. *DH*: Folic acid 400 mcg *SH*: Lives with boyfriend, teacher. Non-smoker, no alcohol intake. *Information*: Had positive pregnancy test 2 weeks ago. Noticed some bleeding yesterday. You are a locum GP.	*PC*: *"I am really worried as I'm pregnant and have been bleeding".* *HPC*: Still bleeding now. Has changed pad 2x this morning. **LMP 6 weeks ago. Abdominal pain since this morning – mostly in right lower abdomen. Moderate severity.** Trying to get pregnant for past 8 months. *ICE*: **Worried about a miscarriage.** *O/E*: BP 100/60, HR 110. Temp 36°C. Abdominal exam – moderate tenderness in RIF.

Child health

Nocturnal enuresis

- Nocturnal enuresis is bed-wetting at night in a child aged 5 years or older, in the absence of congenital or acquired defects of the central nervous system or urinary tract.
- Approximately 1 in 7 children aged five, and 1 in 20 children aged ten, wet the bed.
- Primary nocturnal enuresis refers to a child who has never been dry at night, whereas secondary nocturnal enuresis implies that the child had bladder control for a period of 6 months or more before the bed-wetting started.

Data gathering

Open question
- *"Please can you tell me more about your child's bed-wetting?"*

Focused/closed questions

HPC: *"When did the bed-wetting first start?"*
"Has he/she ever been dry at night?"
"How often is the bedwetting occurring?"
"Is he/she ever wetting in the day?"
"Does he/she have any pain when passing urine?"
"Are there any problems with his/her bowels?"
"Any other medical problems?"
"Does he/she drink many fizzy or caffeinated drinks?"
"Does your child avoid using certain toilets, such as school toilets?"
"Has your child been passing more urine than normal or have they had increased thirst?" (red flags)
"Any weight loss?" (red flag)
N.B. Always remember to consider any features of child maltreatment (red flag)

PMH: Any other medical problems?
DH: *"Does your child take any medication?"*
SH: Any problems at home or at school? Bullying?
FH: Any family history of bed-wetting?

ICE: *"Do you have any idea as to what is causing the bed-wetting?"*
       "What were you hoping we could do to help?"

Examination: • Plot growth on centile chart.
                 • Abdominal examination.

Clinical management

Investigations
- Urine dipstick – to check for glucose and leucocytes (only perform if recent onset of bedwetting, daytime symptoms or symptoms/signs suggestive of diabetes or a UTI).
- Bladder diary for fluid in/out over 48 hours and incontinence episodes over 7 days.

Explanation to parent/patient
- Urine is stored in the bladder, which stretches like a balloon as it fills up. When it stretches to a certain point, the nerves in the bladder wall send a message to the brain saying that it needs to be emptied. Urine then passes out through the urethra. If a child is asleep and the brain does not 'hear' this message, the bladder empties anyway.
- There can be many different reasons for bed-wetting including infection, constipation, too many fizzy drinks or it can be due to psychological factors.

Management
(based on *NICE*, 2010, *CG111: Nocturnal enuresis*)
- Patience and reassurance. It is important that the child knows it is not their fault and punitive measures should not be used.
- Do not restrict drinks but avoid caffeinated drinks before bedtime.
- Recommended fluid intake is >1 litre/day for children aged 4–8 years, increasing to 2.5 l/day for teenage girls and 3.2 l/day for teenage boys.
- Make sure your child goes to the toilet before bed, and also leave a bathroom light on so there is no fear about getting up at night.
- Treat constipation or UTI if present.
- Use a waterproof mattress cover.
- Reward system, e.g. a star chart which can be used if the child achieves a set goal.
- Bed-wetting alarm – 'conditions' children to wake and go to the toilet when their bladder is full. First line treatment if bed-wetting has not responded to the above measures.
- Desmopressin – reduces the amount of urine made at night by the kidneys. Offered to those over 7 years if rapid onset of bed-wetting and/or if short term improvement in bed-wetting is the priority of treatment. Trial cessation every 3 months and stop if child becomes dry.
- Psychological therapy.
- Safety net – if problem not improving advise to return to GP.

Role play

Information for doctor	Additional information for role player
Patient: Master JH *Age*: 8 years *PMH*: Nocturnal enuresis *DH*: Nil *FH*: Older brother had nocturnal enuresis *Information*: Last consultation 3 months ago with salaried GP – nocturnal enuresis. Advised to try lifestyle changes and reward system. You are a locum GP.	*PC*: Mum came in today as JH's bed-wetting is no better. *HPC*: **No daytime wetting. No weight loss, increased thirst or passing large amounts of urine. Likes drinking fizzy drinks.** Wet at night 3–4 times weekly. Has had periods of being dry in the past, but for the past 2 years has been bed-wetting. *SH*: Doesn't like school very much. Gets bullied. *ICE*: Would like referral to specialist as he has had this problem for 2 years and it is not getting any better.

Childhood constipation

- Describes either difficulty or straining when passing stools, passing stools less frequently than normal, or passing hard stools.
- Causes include poor diet, inadequate fluid intake, holding stools in, or medical causes such as bowel disorders.
- Constipation in childhood is common and often associated with faecal incontinence.

Data gathering

Open question
- *"Can you tell me more about the problems your child has been having with their bowels?"*

Focused/closed questions
HPC: *"When did the problem first start?"* (constipation since birth is a possible red flag)
"How often does your child open his/her bowels?"
Any straining or pain when opening bowels?
"How would you describe the stools? Hard and large? Rabbit droppings?"
Any blood in the stools? (red flag)
Any soiling?
Any abdominal pain?
"Are there any problems with your child's growth or development?" (red flag)

"Any vomiting or abdominal swelling?" (red flag – could indicate obstruction)

PMH: Any history of bowel problems?

SH: Any problems at home or at school?

DH: Is he/she on any regular medications?

ICE: *"Do you have any thoughts as to what is causing the constipation?"*

Examination:
- Weight and height (plot on growth chart)
- Abdominal examination
- Inspection of skin and anatomical structures of the lumbo-sacral and gluteal region (to rule out neurological disorders, e.g. spina bifida).
- Inspection of anus – to rule out NAI.
- PR examination – should only be undertaken by healthcare professionals competent to interpret features of anatomical abnormalities or Hirschsprung's disease (do not perform in children >1 year of age with a red flag symptom).

Clinical management

Investigations
- TFTs or coeliac antibodies if considering organic cause for constipation.
- Other investigations should only be requested by a specialist.

Explanation to parent
- Constipation is a common problem in childhood.
- It can develop for a number of reasons and does not normally indicate anything physically wrong with your child.
- Treatment can sometimes take months but symptoms do usually improve.

Management
- Dietary advice – high fibre diet, increased fluid intake, fewer fizzy drinks (NICE advises not to use dietary interventions alone as first line treatment).
- Daily physical activity tailored to child's stage of development.
- Behavioural interventions – stool diary, scheduled toileting, reward system.
- Medication – first line is movicol; second line is stimulant laxative, e.g. senna; third line is osmotic laxative, e.g. lactulose if stools still hard. Continue treatment for several weeks after regular bowel habit is established.
- Patient information: patient.info/health/constipation-in-children-leaflet.
- Refer to paediatrics if no response to initial treatment within 3 months (*NICE*, 2010, *CG99: Constipation in children and young people*).

Role play

Information for doctor	Additional information for role player
Patient: Master RB *Age*: 6 years *FH*: Nil *PMH*: Nil *DH*: Nil *Information*: Mum has booked an appointment today to discuss her son RB. You are a locum GP.	*PC*: *"My son hasn't opened his bowels for 6 days"* *HPC*: Recently hard stools, and straining. Problem started 3 months ago. No blood in stools. No abdominal pain or vomiting. No other symptoms. No concerns about growth and development. **Doesn't drink much water – prefers fizzy drinks. Doesn't like fruit. Prefers crisps. Always leaves his vegetables. Not very active. No concerns at home and mum not aware of any problems at school.** *ICE*: Would like medication for his constipation. *O/E*: 75th centile for height and weight. Abdo. exam – NAD.

Attention deficit hyperactivity disorder

- ADHD is a condition affecting behaviour, which usually first presents in childhood, but can also occur in adults.
- Characterised by hyperactivity, impulsiveness and/or inattention.
- Symptoms must be present for at least 6 months, and impairment in social, academic or occupational functioning must be evident in more than one setting.
- Cause is not fully known, although it could be genetic, environmental or related to an antenatal or obstetric problem.
- Management includes multidisciplinary team involvement, methylphenidate or psychological therapy.

Data gathering

Open question
- *"Can you tell me more about your child's behaviour?"*

Focused/closed questions
HPC: *"How long have you had concerns about your child's behaviour?"*
"Is he/she more restless than most other children?"
"Have there been any concerns about him/her at school? How is he/she doing academically?"
"Have you had concerns about his/her concentration/attention at home?"
"Do you have any concerns with his/her development?" (red flag)
FH: Any FH of ADHD?
DH: Does your child take any regular medications?
SH: Does he/she have brothers or sisters at home? How is the interaction at home with his/her siblings?

ICE: *"Do you have any thoughts as to what might be causing the behavioural problems?"*
"How is this behaviour affecting the family?"

Examination: • Height and weight (plot on growth chart)
• BP
• Assess child's behaviour and interaction with family members (always remember to consider any child protection concerns – red flag)

Clinical management

Investigations

- Nothing specific.

Explanation to parent / patient

- ADHD is a common condition affecting behaviour.
- There is no simple test to diagnose ADHD.
- If your child has symptoms suggestive of ADHD, it is likely that they will be referred to a specialist who will be able to confirm the diagnosis by doing an assessment, and start any treatment if necessary.

Management

(based on *NICE, 2008, CG72: Attention deficit hyperactivity disorder*)

- Provide support for family and involve whole family in management (consider family therapy).
- Consider watchful waiting for up to 10 weeks in mild cases. Can offer referral to parent-training/education programme or for cognitive behavioural therapy.
- Behavioural interventions in the classroom at school can be offered if the teacher has received training.
- Encourage balanced diet, good nutrition and regular exercise. Eliminating artificial colouring and additives from the diet is not a recommended treatment.
- If behavioural problems persist refer to secondary care.
- Medication – methylphenidate, atomoxetine or dexamfetamine (N.B. do not diagnose or start drug treatment in primary care).

Role play

Information for doctor	Additional information for role player
Patient: Master TA *Age*: 7 years *FH*: Has 2 brothers aged 9 and 10 years. Eldest brother has ADHD. *PMH*: Nil *DH*: Nil *Information*: You are a salaried GP. Seen in the surgery with his step-father.	*PC*: Hyperactive child, poor attention span. Teacher at school concerned as he is disruptive in class. *HPC*: **Poor concentration. Not doing well at school for past year. Also very difficult to manage at home due to hyperactivity and restlessness.** *ICE*: **Mum worried that he may have ADHD as he has very similar symptoms to his eldest brother.** *O/E*: Height and weight on 50th centile. Developmental examination normal. Behaviour – hyperactive and impulsive.

Diarrhoea and vomiting

- Diarrhoea and vomiting caused by gastroenteritis is common in young children, especially those under 5 years.
- Diarrhoea usually lasts for around 5–7 days and vomiting usually lasts for 1–2 days.
- Most cases can be managed at home with advice from healthcare professionals.
- An oral vaccine against rotavirus infection, a common cause of diarrhoea and vomiting, is given as two doses for babies aged 8 and 12 weeks, alongside their other routine childhood vaccinations. Since its introduction into the vaccination programme, the rotavirus vaccine has prevented more than 70% of cases.

Data gathering

Open question

- *"Can you tell me a bit more about the diarrhoea and vomiting your child has been experiencing?"*

Focused/closed questions

HPC: *"When did the diarrhoea start?"*

"How many times a day has he/she had diarrhoea?"

"Is there any blood in the stools?" (red flag)

"Any mucus in the stools?"

"How many times has your child vomited in the past 24 hours?"

"When did the vomiting start?"

"Any fever?"

"Any tummy pain?"

"How many wet nappies has your child had in the past 24 hours?"

"Is your child able to keep any fluids down?"

"Has your child been feeding ok?"

"Any recent overseas travel?"

"Has your child been more drowsy than usual?" (red flag)

SH: *"Is anyone else unwell at home?"*

ICE: *"What were you hoping we could do to help?"* *"What concerns did you have about your child?"*

Examination:
- Temperature, pulse, RR.
- Assess hydration status – skin turgor, mucous membranes, CRT, check fontanelle in babies.
- Abdominal examination.

N.B. Red flags include drowsiness, dehydration and signs of shock (tachycardia, tachypnoea, hypotension).

Clinical management

(based on *NICE*, 2009, *CG84: Diarrhoea and vomiting*)

Investigations

- Stool microscopy if you suspect septicaemia or if blood or mucus in stool, or if child is immunocompromised. Consider stool microscopy if recent overseas travel or if no improvement after 7 days.

Management

General advice

- Hand washing and avoid sharing towels.
- Avoid school or nursery if your child has diarrhoea or vomiting caused by gastroenteritis (should not return until at least 48 hours since last episode).
- Avoid swimming in pools for 2 weeks after last episode of diarrhoea.
- Notify public health authority if suspected outbreak of gastroenteritis.
- Do not give anti-diarrhoeals and do not routinely give antibiotics.
- Safety net – give parents information on how to recognise red flag symptoms. Refer urgently to secondary care if clinical signs of dehydration or unable to tolerate oral fluids.

In children with gastroenteritis but without clinical dehydration:

- continue breastfeeding and other milk feeds and encourage fluid intake
- avoid drinking fruit juices and carbonated drinks
- offer oral rehydration salt solution to those at increased risk of dehydration
- during rehydration therapy avoid solid foods.

Role play

Information for doctor	Additional information for role player
Patient: Master JK *Age*: 18 months *SH*: Has older brother aged 3 years. *Information*: You are a locum GP. This child has come to the surgery today with his mother as he has had D&V for the past 2 days. His brother has also been unwell with similar symptoms.	*PC*: Mum is worried about son as he has had bad diarrhoea for the past 2 days and this morning started vomiting. *HPC*: 7× daily diarrhoea and 2 episodes of vomiting today. Watery diarrhoea. **No blood or mucus.** No abdominal discomfort. No fever. **Not drinking as much as usual and not eating but keeping some fluids down.** Only 1 wet nappy this morning. *ICE*: Mum thinks he might need anti-diarrhoea medication. *O/E*: Temp 36.8°C, HR 80, RR 40, CRT <2 secs. Moist mucous membranes. Normal skin turgor. Abdo exam NAD.

Wheeze in preschool children (1–5 years)

- Preschool wheeze affects around 25% of children by 18 months of age (*BMJ*, 2014; 348: g15 – *Managing wheeze in preschool children*).
- There are two main types of wheeze – episodic viral wheeze or multiple trigger wheeze.
- Common practice is to use inhaled beta agonists and steroids in either inhaled or oral form.
- Evidence questions the rationale for steroid use, especially as research suggests even moderate doses of inhaled steroids in the young can cause growth suppression.

Data gathering

Open question
- *"What problems has she been having with her breathing?"*

Focused/closed questions

HPC: *"Have you noticed a cough or a wheeze?"*
"Have these symptoms been worse at any particular time of the day?"
"Has he/she been feeding/eating and drinking well?"
"Has he/she had a temperature?"
"Has he/she been unwell recently with a cold/virus?"

PMH: Any previous breathing problems or admissions to hospital?

SH: Anyone smoking at home? Any other family members unwell?

FH: Any family history of asthma or atopy?

ICE: *"What particular concerns did you have?"*

Examination:
- HR, RR, CRT.
- Oxygen saturations.
- Chest examination.

Clinical management

Investigations
- Blood test – check eosinophil count if appropriate (raised in multiple trigger wheeze).

Explanation to patient
- Wheezing is a whistling sound that occurs during breathing when the airways are narrowed.
- Wheeze is a very common symptom that can occur with a wide range of lung and airways disorders at any age.

- Two common causes of wheeze are asthma and viral infections.
- One type of wheeze in preschool children is called episodic viral wheeze. This type of wheeze only occurs with viral upper respiratory infections and you don't get symptoms in between.
- Another type of wheeze is multiple trigger wheeze. This occurs with upper respiratory tract infections but also with other triggers such as cigarette smoke, exercise and allergic triggers.

Management

Episodic wheeze

- Optimise home environment – no smoking!
- Intermittent bronchodilator (short acting beta agonist or anticholinergic) during wheezy episodes via spacer.
- If symptoms not controlled:
  - add intermittent leukotriene receptor antagonist (montelukast) *or*
  - add intermittent inhaled corticosteroids *or*
  - add both of above.
- No benefit in prophylactic inhaled corticosteroids for majority
  - Consider trial of 6–8 weeks if very severe episodic wheeze then discontinue and review.
- Prednisolone no benefit in children well enough to be managed in the community.

Multiple trigger wheeze

- Intermittent treatment as per episodic wheeze.
- Consider trial of preventative treatment in children with wheeze or cough responsive to bronchodilators plus breathlessness most days, even when no infection is present:
  - trial inhaled corticosteroids or leukotriene receptor antagonist for 4–8 weeks
  - stop treatment
    - if no improvement consider referral for further investigation
    - if symptoms have improved use lowest beneficial dose.

Role play

Information for doctor	Additional information for role player
Patient: Miss KA *Age:* 3 years *PMH:* Nil *DH:* Nil *Information:* You are a salaried GP. Mrs RA has come in to see you with her daughter and is concerned about her breathing.	*PC:* "I'm worried about my daughter as she has had a terrible cough and is very wheezy at night". *HPC:* Cough on and off for past 6 weeks. Runny nose for past couple of weeks. Wheezing mainly past 2–3 nights and not improving. **Intermittent fever. Dad smokes in the home.** *ICE:* **Worried about asthma.** *O/E:* 37.8°C. RR 50. O$_2$ sats 98% Chest –bilateral wheeze audible, no crackles, coryzal.

Care of older adults

Dementia

- Neurological condition causing a gradual loss of mental ability.
- It can also cause changes in personality, decline in social function and a decline in the ability to look after oneself.
- 75% of patients with dementia experience non-cognitive BPSD (behavioural and psychological symptoms of dementia). These may include hallucinations, delusions, and anxiety. Behaviour that challenges may include aggression, agitation, wandering, hoarding, sexual disinhibition, and shouting.
- The most common cause of dementia is Alzheimer's disease, although other types include vascular dementia and Lewy body dementia.
- About 1 in 5 people over the age of 80 have dementia.
- Early diagnosis is important to initiate support and allow advanced planning. Primary care plays a key role in this through opportunistic assessment of at-risk patients and excluding potentially treatable reversible causes, such as depression, thyroid dysfunction and Vitamin B_{12} deficiency.
- There is no cure, although some medications can help to slow the decline in symptoms.

Data gathering

Open question
- *"What can you tell me about the memory problems you have been experiencing?"*

Focused/closed questions

HPC: *"When did you first start to notice problems with your memory?"*
"Were these changes very sudden?" (red flag)
"Is there anything in particular that you forget, for example, names, places, dates?"
"Do you have difficulty with your short term memory, long term memory or both?"
"What is your concentration like?"
"Has anyone noticed any change in your personality or mood?"
"Did you have a fall or head injury?" (red flag)

PMH: Any relevant medical conditions? Any previous operations?

DH: *"Do you take any regular medications?"*

FH: Any family history of dementia or memory problems?

SH: Who lives with you at home? Support? Any carers? Smoking/alcohol/ illicit drug history?

ICE: *"What concerns do you have with your memory?"*

"How has this problem been impacting on your daily life?"

Examination:
- Neurological examination.
- Cognitive assessment via GPCOG (a score of <4 in Section 1 indicates cognitive impairment; a score of 5–8 is indeterminate and triggers an informant questionnaire from a relative, which can be done over the phone) (see *Appendix 3*).
- Mental capacity assessment (if appropriate).

Clinical management
(based on *NICE*, 2011, *CG42: Dementia*)

Investigation
- Dementia blood screen – FBC, U&Es, LFTs, calcium, glucose, folate, B_{12} and TFTs.
- Urinalysis – to rule out UTI.
- MRI brain (or alternatively CT) – refer to memory clinic first.

Explanation to patient
- Alzheimer's disease is the commonest type of dementia.
- It is caused by shrinkage of the brain, resulting in a reduction in the number of nerve fibres.
- The levels of some brain chemicals called neurotransmitters are also reduced, in particular acetylcholine, although the reason for this leading to memory problems is not clearly understood.
- Tiny deposits or plaques also form within the brain which can damage surrounding nerve cells. They can spread to the hippocampus part of the brain which is essential in forming memories.

Management
- Refer to memory clinic for further assessment and investigations.
- Provide written information about dementia and the local care and support services available.
- Support and care from community teams, for example, district nurses, psychiatric teams, occupational therapy and social services.
- Physical activity and cognitive group stimulation programme (for those with mild dementia).
- Treat any risk factors for dementia, for example, smoking, excessive alcohol use, obesity, hypertension and high cholesterol.
- Develop individualised care plan and review regularly – important to retain familiar environment, consistent and stable staffing, and minimise relocations.
- Medication is usually started by specialist and includes acetylcholinesterase inhibitors (e.g. donepezil, galantamine) in mild–moderate Alzheimer's disease (MMSE score 10–20). Memantine (NMDA antagonist) can be used for moderate to severe Alzheimer's dementia.

- Consider medication for non-cognitive symptoms or behaviour that challenges in the first instance only if there is severe distress or an immediate risk of harm to the person with dementia or others.
- Inform DVLA if still driving.
- Consider whether the patient has capacity to make decisions about their care. If the person lacks capacity, the provisions of the Mental Capacity Act 2005 must be followed (*NICE*, 2011, *CG42: Dementia*).
- Consider the carer's needs.
- Safety net – if problems worsen to return to GP.

Role play

Information for doctor	Additional information for role player
Patient: Mrs WW *Age*: 83 years *SH*: Lives with husband. Non-smoker. No alcohol. *FH*: Nil *PMH*: MI 1996, hypercholesterolaemia *DH*: Aspirin 75 mg OD, simvastatin 40 mg nocte. *Information*: You are a GP partner. Mr W has booked an appointment to chat about his wife.	*PC*: *"I am worried about my wife as she seems to be getting increasingly confused"* *HPC*: Gradual deterioration in memory over past 9 months. Was found wandering the streets last week. **Gets confused with where she is, and days of the week.** Still has good long-term memory. Last week she left her gas hob on. No aggression or low mood. *ICE*: **Worried she may be developing Alzheimer's.** *O/E*: Neurological examination – NAD. MMSE – 14/30.

Falls

- Common presentation in the elderly, often with multi-factorial aetiology.
- After a hip fracture 40% end up in institutional care, 20% never walk again and 30% die within a year.
- Risk factors include previous falls history, gait and balance problems, home hazards, visual impairment, cognitive impairment, muscle weakness, hypotension and poly-pharmacy.
- Management depends on the cause, although the NICE guidelines (2013, *CG161: Falls in older people*) advise multi-factorial interventions.

Data gathering

Open question
- *"Can you tell me more about the falls you've been experiencing?"*

Focused/closed questions
HPC: *"How frequently are you having these falls?"*
"Do you know what is causing the falls?"
"Have you ever lost consciousness?"
"Have you ever injured yourself?"

"Do you get any associated dizziness beforehand?"
Were there any witnesses?
"Have you ever experienced the sensation of your heart pounding?"
"Have you ever lost control of your bladder?"

PMH: Any medical conditions?

FH: Any FH of osteoporosis or falls?

SH: *"Who lives with you at home?"* *"Do you have stairs at home?"* Support? Coping? Alcohol history?

DH: *"Are you on any regular medications?"* *"Do you take any blood pressure medications/sedatives?"*

Examination: (includes multifactorial falls risk assessment – *NICE, 2004, CG21: Falls*):

- BP, pulse.
- BMI.
- Cardiovascular system.
- Neurological examination including visual acuity, gait, mobility and balance.
- Timed up and go test – record the time it takes your patient to rise from a chair, walk 3 metres (using their usual mobility aid), turn round, walk back to the chair and sit down. >30 secs suggests a more significant falls risk.
- Assessment of cognitive impairment.

ICE: *"Do you fear falling at home?"*

Clinical management

Investigations

- Blood test – FBC, U&Es, LFTs, TFTs, B_{12}, glucose.
- Urinalysis – check for leucocytes and nitrites.
- ECG.
- DEXA scan – if at risk of osteoporosis.

Explanation to patient

- There are lots of different risk factors for falls. These include low body weight, being on medications such as beta-blockers and insulin, alcohol abuse, diabetes mellitus, confusion, and problems with vision or balance.
- There are various different measures which can be taken to help prevent falls.

Management

- Consider falls clinic.
- Multifactorial intervention – stop any causative medications, strength and balance training, home hazard assessment and intervention, management of any visual problems, assess osteoporosis risk, walking aids. Podiatry – in people with disabling foot pain. Cataract surgery – in people with cataracts.
- Provide information leaflet about falls prevention (there are great resources from STEADI on how to stay independent).
- Safety net – arrange follow-up to assess progress.

Role play

Information for doctor	Additional information for role player
Patient: Mrs VH	*PC*: Falls
Age: 84 years	*HPC*: Has had several falls in recent weeks and
SH: Lives alone in warden-controlled flat.	the warden is quite concerned. Episodes of
PMH: Previous mitral valve repair 2006,	dizziness. **No syncope. No palpitations or**
hypertension, hypothyroidism.	**SOB. No loss of consciousness. Warden**
DH: Coracten XL 30 mg OD, levothyroxine	**witnessed one fall. Seemed to lose balance.**
50 mcg OD, aspirin 75 mg OD.	No known triggers. **Has had bruising and**
Information: Was seen by the practice nurse for	**cut to head. Had recent eye test which was**
BP check last week (100/60 mmHg).	**satisfactory.**
Mentioned to nurse about recent	*ICE*: Warden concerned about the falls.
history of falls. You are a salaried GP.	*O/E*: Sitting BP 120/80, standing BP 80/50. CVS
	exam NAD. HR 70, regular. Neuro exam NAD.
	Gait – unsteady.

Women's health

Menorrhagia

- Heavy periods, often defined as blood loss >80 mls.
- Cause is often not known, and this is referred to as 'dysfunctional uterine bleeding'.
- Other causes include fibroids, endometriosis, IUD *in situ* or hypothyroidism.
- Management includes LNG-IUS, tranexamic acid, COCP or surgical options.

Data gathering

Open question

- *"Can you tell me more about the heavy periods that you've been experiencing?"*

Focused/closed questions

HPC: *"When did the heavy periods first start?"*
"Was the heavy bleeding sudden in onset?" (red flag)
"How many times do you change pads/tampons in a typical day?"
"Do you get any clots in the blood or any flooding?"
"Are your periods more painful than usual?"
"Do you get any abdominal pain or abdominal bloating?"
"Are your periods regular? When was your last menstrual period?"
"Do you get any bleeding in between your periods or after sex?" (red flag)
"Are you using any contraception at present? If so, what?"
"When was your last smear test?"
"Any abnormal discharge or risks of any sexually transmitted infections?"

PMH: Any other medical conditions? Any previous gynaecological surgery? Any previous pregnancies?

DH: *"Are you on any regular medications?"* (specifically enquire about aspirin and anticoagulants)

FH: Any conditions that run in the family? Any bleeding disorders?

ICE: *"Do you have any thoughts as to what might be causing the heavy bleeding?"*
"How is this problem affecting your day to day life?"

Examination:
- Abdominal/pelvic examination (red flags include pelvic mass and features of PID).
- Speculum examination (take swabs if infection is suspected).
N.B. Offer chaperone.

Clinical management

Investigations

- Blood tests – FBC, TFTs (only if symptomatic), clotting screen (if suggestive features in the history).
- Vaginal/endocervical swabs for MC&S and STI screen (if at risk).
- Ultrasound scan of pelvis (if concerned about structural abnormality).

Explanation to patient

- Heavy periods often occur because the amount of a chemical called prostaglandin is increased in the lining of the womb.
- It can also be caused by fibroids (benign growths in the womb), endometriosis (endometrial tissue grows outside the womb) or a hormonal problem.

Management

- Menstrual diary.
- LNG-IUS (Mirena) – reduces heavy menstrual bleeding (NICE first line).
- Consider urgent referral to gynaecology if suspicious mass is detected.
- Medications – tranexamic acid, COCP, norethisterone.
- Safety net – to see GP if problem not improving.
- Surgery – endometrial ablation, hysterectomy.

Role play

Information for doctor	Additional information for role player
Patient: Ms JE *Age*: 26 years *SH*: PhD student, lives with partner *PMH*: migraine *DH*: Nil *FH*: Nil *Information*: You are a GP Registrar.	*PC*: *"I have been getting very heavy periods for the past 6 months"* *HPC*: Period lasts 7 days. Changing tampons approx every 3 hours. **Has clots. No flooding.** Regular periods (LMP 2 weeks ago). Also gets quite severe abdominal pain during periods. **No discharge. No IMB/PCB. Has copper IUD *in situ*** (fitted 8 months ago). *ICE*: Would like some medication to help reduce the heavy bleeding. Also keen to know what is causing it. *O/E*: Abdominal examination – lower abdominal tenderness. Slight tenderness on PV examination.

Amenorrhoea

- Absence or cessation of menses, either classified as primary amenorrhoea (menses not occurring by the time of expected menarche) or secondary amenorrhoea (absence of menstruation for at least 6 consecutive months in women with previously normal and regular menses).
- Causes of primary amenorrhoea include constitutional delay, genito-urinary malformation, Turner syndrome and testicular feminisation.

- Causes of secondary amenorrhoea include hypothalamic failure, pregnancy and lactation, premature ovarian failure, weight loss, polycystic ovarian syndrome and depot or implant contraception.

Data gathering

Open question
- *"Can you tell me more about the problem with your periods?"*

Focused/closed questions

HPC: *"Have you ever had periods? If so, when was your last menstrual period?"*
"At what age did you start having periods (if secondary amenorrhoea)?"
"Is there any chance you could be pregnant?" *"Are you sexually active at present?"* *"What are you currently using for contraception?"* (if relevant)
"Have there been any recent change in your weight or any increase in exercise?"
"Have you been more stressed than usual recently?"
"Have you noticed any changes to your skin or hair?"
"Any lower abdominal pain?" (haematocolpos)
"Any hot flushes or vaginal dryness?" (menopause/premature ovarian failure)
"Have you ever had problems trying to get pregnant?"
"Any headache, problems with your vision or leakage of milk from your breasts?" (red flags)

PMH: Any medical conditions? PCOS? Thyroid problems? Depression? Eating disorders? Previous surgery?

DH: *"Do you take any regular medications?"* Any hormonal contraceptives? Antipsychotics? Previous radiotherapy or chemotherapy? Steroids?

FH: Any family history of menstrual problems? *"When did your mother and sister(s) start their periods?"*
Any family history of stopping periods before 40 years of age?

SH: Occupation/Studying? Stress? Who lives with you at home? Any problems? Illicit drug use, e.g. cocaine or opiates?

ICE: *"Do you have any thoughts as to why your periods might have stopped?"*

Examination
(based on NHS CKS, 2014, Amenorrhoea – management):
- BMI, BP.
- Examine for secondary sexual characteristics, e.g. Tanner Stages (N.B. no intimate examinations in the CSA).
- Examine for hirsutism, clitoromegaly, galactorrhoea and haematocolpos (if appropriate from history).
- Thyroid examination (if appropriate from history).
- Visual fields/fundoscopy (if pituitary tumour suspected).
- Cranial nerve examination.
- Pelvic examination – only in older women if appropriate.

Clinical management

Investigations
- Pregnancy test.
- Blood tests – serum LH, FSH, prolactin, glucose, TSH, testosterone, SHBG.
- Pelvic ultrasound scan.
- If suspecting a prolactinoma refer to secondary care for an MRI of the brain.

Explanation to patient
- Amenorrhoea is the absence of menstrual periods in a woman of reproductive age.
- There may be a normal physiological explanation, for example, before puberty or due to pregnancy, breast-feeding or menopause, or it may be due to contraception, surgery or due to a medical condition.

Management
(based on *NHS CKS*, 2014, *Amenorrhoea – management*)

Primary amenorrhoea
- Refer to a specialist any female who has not started menstruating by 14 years of age and has no secondary sexual characteristics, or females with normal secondary sexual characteristics who have not started menstruating by 16 years of age.

Secondary amenorrhoea
- Treat the underlying cause once the diagnosis is confirmed, e.g. counselling if stress induced or stopping any causative drugs.
- Refer to a specialist if the cause cannot be established or if treatment in secondary care is required.
- The following conditions can usually be managed in primary care – PCOS, menopause and amenorrhoea due to weight loss, stress or exercise.
- Manage the risk of osteoporosis.
- Safety net – if not resolving to return to GP.

Role play

Information for doctor	Additional information for role player
Patient: Ms SL *Age*: 17 years *SH*: College student, lives with parents. Non-smoker. No alcohol or illicit drug use. *PMH*: Acne *DH*: Nil *Information*: Consultation with locum GP 2 weeks ago – tiredness, weight gain. TFTs checked and normal. BMI 34. You are a GP partner.	*PC*: "*I have not had a period for the past 8 months*". *HPC*: Previously had periods. Started menstruating aged 12 years. Also increased facial hair. No skin changes. No headache or visual problems. 6 kg weight gain in past 6 months. **Sexually active – uses condoms.** No abdo pain. No milk leakage from breasts. **Recent stress due to exams.** *FH:* **No menstrual problems.** *ICE:* **Worried about being pregnant. Hoping for a pregnancy test.** *O/E:* Pregnancy test – negative. Evidence of hirsutism.

Premenstrual syndrome

- Condition in which women experience certain symptoms each month before their menstrual period.
- Most commonly affects women aged between 30 and 40 years.
- Symptoms may be physical (e.g. breast tenderness, bloating, headaches) and/or psychological (e.g. tension, irritability, low mood, loss of libido).
- Treatments include SSRIs, COCP or CBT.

Data gathering

Open question
- *"Can you describe the symptoms you experience prior to your period?"*

Focused/closed questions

HPC: *"Do you suffer with any breast tenderness, bloating or headaches prior to your period?"*
"Do you experience any mood changes prior to your period?"
"Have you noticed any changes to your sex drive?"
"How long have you been experiencing these symptoms?"
"How long do they last for each time?"
"When in your cycle do you experience these symptoms?"
"Have you tried anything so far to relieve the symptoms?"
"Are you using any hormonal contraceptives?"

PMH: Any history of depression or any other medical conditions?

DH: *"Do you take any regular medications?"*

FH: Any family history of PMS?

SH: Occupation? Who lives with you at home? Smoking/alcohol/illicit drug history?

ICE: *"How have the symptoms been affecting your day to day life?"*

Examination: • Nothing specific.

Clinical management

Investigations
- Symptom diary (for two or three cycles and then review the woman with the diary).

Explanation to patient
- PMS is quite a common problem, although it is only bad enough to affect daily life in about 1 in 20 women.
- There is no test for PMS and it is diagnosed purely on the symptoms described.
- The cause is not known, although ovulation with the release of an egg appears to trigger symptoms.

Management

(based on *NICE, 2014, CKS: Premenstrual syndrome.*)

- General advice about exercise, diet, stopping smoking, reducing alcohol intake, regular sleep, and stress reduction.
- Medications, e.g. new generation COC for moderate PMS, NSAIDs if pain is predominant problem or SSRI if severe PMS.
- Complementary therapy may be beneficial but studies are limited, e.g. reflexology, evening primrose oil, vitamin B6 from day 14 to menses, magnesium, calcium and agnus castus.
- CBT.
- Information leaflet.
- Safety net – refer to gynaecologist when simple measures have been explored but have failed.

Role play

Information for doctor	Additional information for role player
Patient: Ms TB *Age*: 21 years *SH*: University student. Lives in shared student flat. Smokes 10 cigs/day. Alcohol 30 units/week. *FH*: Nil *PMH*: Nil. No history of depression. *DH*: Nil *Information*: You are a GP partner. Temporary patient.	*PC*: *"I have terrible mood swings around the time of my period".* *HPC*: *"Something needs to be done because I got into trouble in a night club last weekend as I got aggressive towards someone".* Also broke up with boyfriend because of aggression/mood. Gets occasional breast tenderness and bloating. No headaches. Has had symptoms for past year. Symptoms start 10 days before period. *ICE*: **Needs some medication to take around her periods to help with mood.**

Polycystic ovary syndrome

- Condition resulting in tiny cysts forming on the ovaries (at least 12 cysts).
- Can result in abnormal periods, reduced fertility, excessive hair growth and acne.
- Exact cause is unclear, but could be hereditary or linked to insulin resistance and/or obesity.
- Treatment depends on the symptoms, but includes weight loss, metformin and/or hormonal contraception to regulate periods.
- The figure on the next page shows how you could illustrate polycystic ovaries to your patient.

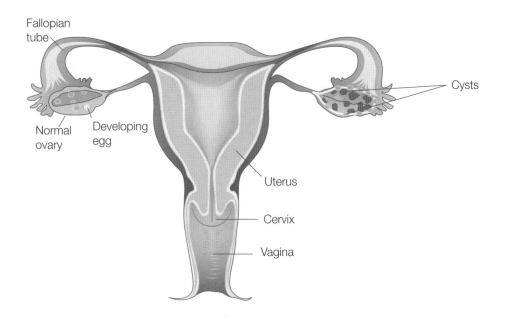

Fallopian tube

Cysts

Normal ovary

Developing egg

Uterus

Cervix

Vagina

Data gathering

Open questions

- *"What do you know about polycystic ovary syndrome?"*
- *"Can you tell me more about your symptoms?"*

Focused/closed questions

HPC: *"When was your last menstrual period?"*
"Are your periods regular? Have there been any changes in your periods recently?"
"Do you get any abdominal pain?"
"Have you noticed any skin changes or excessive hair growth?"
"Have there been any changes in your mood?"
"Have there been any changes in your weight?"
"Any problems trying to get pregnant?"

PMH: *"Have you had any obstetric or gynaecological problems in the past?"*

FH: Any family history of PCOS?

SH Smoking/alcohol/illicit drug history? Occupation? Stress?

ICE: *"Was there anything in particular you were concerned about with these symptoms?"* (common concerns include fertility and self esteem issues)

Examination:
- BMI.
- BP.
- Examination for acne and hirsutism.
- Pelvic examination.

Clinical management

Investigations

- Blood test – total and free testosterone, SHBG, free androgen index, prolactin, TSH*.
- Glucose tolerance test – if symptoms suggestive of PCOS, obese or FH of diabetes.
- Pregnancy test (if appropriate).
- Pelvic ultrasound scan.

*LH and FSH are not routinely recommended for diagnosis of PCOS, but may help to rule out other causes (*RCOG*, 2007, *Green-top guideline 33: Long term consequences of polycystic ovary syndrome*).

Explanation to patient

- PCOS is a condition which can affect a woman's menstrual cycle, fertility, hormones and aspects of her appearance. It can also affect long-term health.
- Cysts develop on the ovaries which results in an imbalance of the hormones produced by the ovaries.
- The ovaries produce more testosterone which can result in excessive hair growth and acne. The hormones released by the ovary are responsible for controlling the menstrual cycle and so this can also be affected.
- Some patients may no longer ovulate which will result in fertility problems.

Management

- Lifestyle changes – weight loss, healthy balanced diet, exercise and smoking cessation.
- Metformin (topic for debate but not recommended for initiation in primary care. Recent RCTs have not shown metformin to reduce weight or restore menstrual regularity in women with PCOS).
- Co-cyprindiol (Dianette) – if symptoms of acne or hirsutism.
- Other hormonal contraceptives to regulate periods.
- Hirsutism – hair removal creams, electrolysis, laser treatment, or eflornithine.
- Fertility problems – clomiphene can be beneficial but refer to gynaecology first.
- Offer annual fasting glucose/HbA1C, fasting lipids and BP.
- In pregnancy check GTT before 20 weeks' gestation.
- Safety net – refer to a specialist if the above measures are not improving symptoms.

Role play

Information for doctor	Additional information for role player
Patient: Ms SS *Age*: 23 years *PMH*: Nil *DH*: Nil *SH*: Non-smoker. Waitress. *Information*: Saw locum GP 1 month ago due to secondary amenorrhoea and hirsutism. USS of pelvis confirms polycystic ovaries. You are a GP Registrar.	*PC*: "*I have come today to get the results of my ultrasound scan*." *HPC*: LMP 8 months ago. Has noticed increased facial hair. **No skin changes. No abdominal pain and no mood changes. No other gynaecological symptoms. Never tried to conceive.** *FH*: **Sister has PCOS.** *ICE*: Thinks that she might also have PCOS. Would like medication to get rid of the increased facial hair. *O/E*: BMI – 34. BP 130/70. Abdo exam – mild lower abdominal tenderness. No masses.

Fibroids

- Benign growths in the uterus.
- Very common, affecting at least 1 in 4 women in their lifetime.
- Commonest in the 30–50 year age group and in Afro–Caribbean women.
- Symptoms only occur in about one-third of women with fibroids.
- Can be treated with medication, LNG-IUS or with surgery.
- The figure below shows how you could illustrate fibroids to your patient.

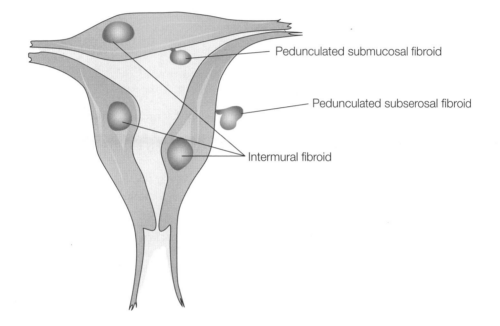

Pedunculated submucosal fibroid

Pedunculated subserosal fibroid

Intermural fibroid

Data gathering

Open questions
- *"Can you tell me more about your symptoms?"*
- *"The recent ultrasound scan you had has confirmed fibroids: what do you know about fibroids?"*

Closed/focused questions
HPC: *"Are your periods regular?"*

"Are your periods heavier than usual?"

"Any bleeding in between your periods or after sex?" (red flags)

"Have you noticed any abdominal pain or swelling?"

"Have you experienced any back pain?"

"Have you experienced any pain during sexual intercourse?"

> "Do you have any urinary symptoms?"
> "Has there been any weight loss?" (red flag)

FH: Any family history of fibroids?

SH: Smoking/alcohol/illicit drug history? Occupation?

ICE: "What were you hoping we could do to help with your symptoms?"

Examination:
- Abdominal examination.
- Vaginal examination.
- Speculum examination – to rule out other causes, e.g. cervical pathology, STI.

Clinical management

Investigations

- Pelvic ultrasound scan.
- FBC – if concerned about anaemia.
- Hysteroscopy or laparoscopy – in secondary care.

Explanation to patient

- Fibroids are non-cancerous growths which form in the womb, usually as a result of an overgrowth of smooth muscle cells.
- They can cause symptoms such as heavy bleeding, abdominal swelling and urinary problems.
- They can increase or decrease in size with time. During pregnancy they often increase in size due to the increased level of a hormone called oestrogen.

Management

- Observation and safety net – if symptoms not improving return to GP.
- Medication – tranexamic acid, NSAIDs, COCP, GnRH analogue to shrink the fibroids.
- LNG-IUS (Mirena) – can be difficult to insert into uterus when fibroids present.
- Referral to secondary care if fibroids are large (>3 cm) or if symptoms not improving despite medication. Further treatment options include endometrial ablation, uterine artery embolisation, hysterectomy, and myomectomy.

Role play

Information for doctor	Additional information for role player
Patient: Mrs JS *Age*: 34 years *PMH*: Nil. No previous pregnancies. *DH*: Ibuprofen 400 mg TDS/PRN *SH*: Non-smoker, no alcohol intake. Teacher. *Information*: Recently seen by locum GP due to abdominal pain and menorrhagia. Results of pelvic USS – numerous fibroids visible in endometrium. Largest 5 cm × 4 cm diameter. You are a GP partner.	*PC*: "I was asked to come in to discuss the results of my pelvic ultrasound scan". *HPC*: Lower abdominal pain for the past couple of months. Also heavy periods. LMP 2 weeks ago. Regular periods. No urinary symptoms. No abdominal swelling. No weight loss. *ICE*: **Worried she might have cancer.** *O/E*: Lower abdominal tenderness. Abdomen soft. No masses palpable. PV exam – slightly bulky uterus.

Antenatal check

- All pregnant women in the UK are offered a series of antenatal appointments during their pregnancy.
- In the case of an uncomplicated pregnancy, this care should be provided by midwives and GPs (*NICE*, 2008, *CG62: Antenatal care*).
- In an uncomplicated pregnancy, nulliparous women are offered 10 antenatal appointments, and parous women are offered 7 appointments.
- The first booking appointment is around 10–12 weeks.
- The antenatal checks include weight, blood pressure, urine dipstick for protein, glucose and leucocytes, and blood tests for blood group, rhesus group and infections.
- The growth of the baby is checked using symphysis–fundal height (SFH), and the position of the baby is also checked in the later stages of pregnancy.
- Ultrasound scans are carried out at 12 and 20 weeks gestation, and screening tests for Down syndrome, sickle cell diseases and thalassaemias are also offered.
- Some women require additional care during pregnancy, including those with cardiac conditions, insulin dependent diabetes, epilepsy or if BMI <18 or >30.

Data gathering

Open question

- *"How is the pregnancy going so far?"*

Focused/closed questions

HPC: *"When was your last menstrual period?"*
"When is your expected date of delivery?"
"Are you getting any abdominal pains?" (red flag)
"Have you noticed any vaginal bleeding?" (red flag)
"Have you felt any kicks or the baby moving?" (only relevant from approximately 20 weeks gestation)
"Do you have any ankle swelling?" (mainly occurs in the latter stages of pregnancy)
"Any history or concerns of domestic violence in the household?" (red flag ; see *Appendix 7*)

PMH: *"Do you suffer from any medical conditions?"* *"Any previous pregnancies?"* *"Any previous pregnancy complications?"* *"Any previous gynaecological problems?"* *"Any mental health problems?"* (red flag)

FH: *"Any medical conditions which run in the family?"*

DH: Do you take any regular medications?
"Have you been taking folic acid?"

SH: Who lives with you at home? Support? Occupation? Smoking/alcohol/illicit drug history?

ICE: *"Do you have any concerns about the pregnancy?"*

Examination: • See clinical management.

Clinical management

(based on *NICE*, 2008, *CG62: Antenatal care*)

First contact with a healthcare professional

- Provide information on folic acid supplements, lifestyle advice and antenatal screening.

Lifestyle advice

- Smoking cessation – nicotine replacement therapy can be used in pregnancy.
- Alcohol consumption – avoid alcohol in the first 3 months if at all possible. If women choose to drink alcohol, drink no more than 1–2 units of alcohol once or twice a week.
- Folic acid supplement prior to conception until 12 weeks gestation – 400 mcg daily (or 5 mg daily if your risk of having a child with a neural tube defect is increased, e.g. coeliac disease, diabetes or if taking anti-convulsants).
- Vitamin D supplements during pregnancy and breast-feeding if inadequate stores – 10 mcg daily.
- Dietary advice – avoid uncooked meat, fish and eggs (toxoplasmosis), liver (vitamin A), soft cheeses and pâté (listeria) and unpasteurised milk. Restrict caffeine intake to no more than 200 mg daily (2 mugs of instant coffee or tea).
- Advise on which drugs to avoid, e.g. NSAIDs.
- Exercise – encourage gentle exercise (avoid contact sports).

Management of nausea and morning sickness

- Very common in the early weeks of pregnancy and can happen at any time of the day (usually disappears around 12th to 14th week).
- Try eating dry toast or a plain biscuit before getting up in the morning.
- Eat small amounts often.
- Drink plenty of fluids.
- Avoid greasy and spicy foods.
- Antihistamines, e.g. metoclopramide.
- Ginger and P6 acupressure may be beneficial.
- Consider hyperemesis gravidarum if persistent vomiting.

Booking appointment

- Identify women who may need additional care.
- Calculate BMI.
- Measure BP and check urine for proteinuria and leucocytes.
- Offer blood test for blood group, rhesus D status, FBC, haemoglobinopathies, Hep B, HIV, rubella immunity and syphilis.
- Offer screening for Down syndrome.
- Offer ultrasound scans for gestational age assessment at 12 weeks and to check for any fetal anomalies at 20 weeks.
- Inform women under 25 years about the national chlamydia screening programme.

- Determine if any risk factors for gestational diabetes* or pre-eclampsia.
- Inform women about maternity benefits available, e.g. free prescriptions and dental care during pregnancy and 12 months after.

*Gestational diabetes

- Risk factors include BMI >30, previous macrosomic baby weighing >4.5 kg, previous gestational diabetes, family history of diabetes or a family origin with a high incidence of diabetes.
- The 2 hour 75 g oral glucose tolerance test (OGTT) should be offered to pregnant women at risk at 24–28 weeks of gestation (or earlier if previous gestational diabetes).

25 weeks (nulliparous women)

- Measure BP and check urine for proteinuria.
- Measure symphysis–fundal height (SFH).

28–34 weeks

- Check SFH.
- Offer pertussis (whooping cough) vaccine – was introduced to pregnant women as part of a temporary programme from October 2012.
- Offer further screening for anaemia.
- Offer anti-D prophylaxis for those women who are rhesus D negative.
- Discuss a birth plan.

36–38 weeks

- Check position of baby, and refer for external cephalic version if breech.
- Discuss breast-feeding and postnatal care.

41 weeks

- If not yet given birth, refer for membrane sweep and induction of labour.

Travel

- Wear car seat belts above and below bump rather than over it.
- There is an increased risk of DVT if flying – wear compression hosiery for long haul flights where possible.
- Discuss vaccinations and travel insurance if travelling abroad.
- Most airlines will not allow women to travel if >36 weeks pregnant (>32 weeks if multiple pregnancies).
- Airlines may require a certificate after 28 weeks stating the pregnancy is progressing normally.
- Most airlines will also not allow women to travel if history of premature delivery, cervical incompetence or PV bleeding.

Role play

Information for doctor	Additional information for role player
Patient: Mrs SC *Age*: 32 years *PMH*: Nil *SH*: Married, Store manager. Non-smoker. No alcohol intake. *DH*: Pregnancy multivitamins *FH*: Nil *Information*: Has appointment today for routine 30 week antenatal check. You are a GP Registrar. Uncomplicated pregnancy so far.	*HPC*: Currently 30 weeks pregnant. Hasn't felt baby moving for the past 24 hours. No vaginal bleeding or abdominal pain. First pregnancy. 20 week scan – NAD. *ICE*: **A bit worried that she hasn't felt fetal movements.** *O/E*: BP 100/60. Urine dip – NAD . SFH 26 cm, no fetal heart sounds heard.

Urinary incontinence

- Involuntary leakage of urine, estimated to affect about 3 million people in the UK.
- Different types include stress, urge, mixed and overflow incontinence.
- Management includes lifestyle changes, pelvic floor exercises, bladder training or medication.

Data gathering

Open question

- "Can you tell me more about the problems with your bladder?"

Closed/focused questions

HPC: *"How often do you lose control of your bladder?" "Is it only when coughing or sneezing, or does it occur at any time?"*
"Are you incontinent in the day and night?"
"Have you tried any treatments so far?"
"Do you suffer with frequent urine infections?"
"Do you have any burning pain when you pass urine?"
"Have you noticed any blood in the urine or vaginal bleeding?" (red flag)
"Have you noticed a lump coming down from your vagina?"
"Do you have any problems with your bowels?"
"How many cups of tea or coffee do you drink daily?" "Any other caffeine intake?"
"How much do you drink in the evening?"

DH: Do you take any regular medications? Diuretics?

FH: Any family history of bladder problems? Any weight loss? (red flag)

SH: Smoking/alcohol/illicit drug history? Occupation?

PMH:	Any previous operations? *"Any previous obstetric problems or urinary problems?"*
ICE:	*"How is this problem impacting on your daily life?"*
Examination:	• Abdominal examination – to check for masses and any enlargement of bladder or kidneys.
	• Digital rectal examination – in males to examine prostate.
	• Sims speculum examination to check for vaginal prolapse.

Clinical management

Investigations

- Urinalysis – blood, glucose, protein, leucocytes, nitrites.
- Urodynamics (only after conservative management).
- U&Es.

Explanation to patient

- There are different types of urinary incontinence:
  - ○ Stress incontinence occurs when the pressure in the bladder becomes too great and urine leaks from the bladder outlet. This is often due to the pelvic floor muscles being weak.
  - ○ Urge incontinence is when you get an urgent desire to pass urine and are unable to get to the toilet in time. It's often due to a problem with the bladder muscles sending wrong messages to the brain.
  - ○ Mixed incontinence is a combination of stress and urge incontinence.
  - ○ Overflow incontinence is due to an obstruction of the outflow of urine.

Management

(*NICE*, 2013, *CG171*: *Urinary incontinence in women*)

Stress incontinence

- Pelvic floor exercises are first line (8 contractions, 3× daily for minimum 3 months).
- If not improving refer if patient wishes.
- Duloxetine may be an option in women preferring to avoid surgery.

Urge incontinence

- Lifestyle advice – reduce caffeine, modify fluid intake, weight loss.
- Bladder retraining.
- Intravaginal oestrogen therapy may be beneficial in post-menopausal women.
- Antimuscarinic drugs, e.g oxybutynin, solifenacin.
- Mirabegron is the new medical option if antimuscarinics are not effective or not tolerated.
- Refer to secondary care for surgical management if conservative management hasn't helped or if there is a symptomatic prolapse visible at or below the vaginal introitus.
- Urgently refer if microscopic haematuria and aged 50 years or over, visible haematuria, suspected pelvic mass arising from the urinary tract or recurrent or persistent UTI associated with haematuria in those aged 40 years or older.

Role play

Information for doctor	Additional information for role player
Patient: Mrs JW *Age*: 47 years *SH*: Married, has 3 children. Alcohol 10 units weekly. *PMH*: Nil *DH*: Nil *Information*: No recent consultations. You are a GP partner.	*PC*: Urinary incontinence *HPC*: Has urinary incontinence intermittently for past 8 months but it is becoming more frequent (now daily). **Occurs mainly after coughing, sneezing or exercise. No blood in the urine. No abdominal pain. No pain when passing urine. Not tried any treatments so far. Two urine infections in the past year.** No constipation or weight loss. **Drinks 4 cups of tea daily. No excessive fluid intake in evening. No dragging sensation down below.** *ICE*: Has heard about surgery to help this problem and is keen to find out more. *O/E*: Abdo exam – NAD. Sims speculum exam – small prolapse of posterior vaginal wall.

Cervical screening

- Offered to all women aged between 25 and 65 in England and Northern Ireland (20–65 years in Scotland and Wales).
- The aim is to detect any pre-cancerous cells.
- The screening is carried out 3-yearly from 20 or 25 years to 50 years and then 5-yearly until aged 65.
- Risk factors for cervical cancer include HPV infection, smoking and immunocompromised states such as HIV.

Data gathering

Open question
- *"What do you understand about an abnormal cervical smear result?"*

Focused/closed questions
HPC: *"Have you had any irregular menstrual bleeding?"*

"Have you had any bleeding in between your periods or after sex?" (red flags)

"Any pain during sexual intercourse?" (red flag)

"Have you noticed any abnormal vaginal discharge?" If so, enquire about colour, consistency and smell.

"Do you have any abdominal pain?"

"Have you recently noticed any weight loss?" (red flag)

"Any urinary symptoms?"

"Are you sexually active at present? If so, do you use condoms?"

"How many sexual partners have you had in the past 3 months?"

"Any past history of sexually transmitted infections?"

PMH: "Any previous abnormal cervical smear tests?"

DH: Current contraceptives?

FH: Any family history of breast cancer, cervical cancer or other gynaecological cancers?

SH: "Do you smoke?" Who lives with you at home? Occupation?

ICE: "Did you have any specific concerns about your smear test result?"

Examination: • Liquid cervical smear test via speculum examination.

Clinical management

Investigations

- Refer for colposcopy if moderate or severe dyskaryosis or two consecutive results showing mild dyskaryosis.

Explanation to patient

- Cells are gently scraped from the neck of the womb using a plastic brush.
- These cells are then sent to the lab to be examined under a microscope.
- If there are any abnormal cells seen, you may be referred for a colposcopy.
- A colposcopy is a detailed examination of the cervix using an instrument called a colposcope. It allows a more detailed view of any abnormal cells in the cervix, and a further sample of tissue can be taken if necessary.
- If the colposcopy reveals an abnormal result, you may need further treatment to remove or destroy the abnormal cells in your cervix. This can be done using laser treatment or by cutting out the affected area. If there are only mild changes in the cervix, the abnormal cells may return to normal on their own.

Management

- Smoking cessation.
- Offer STI screening, if appropriate, and sexual health education.
- Treatment for abnormal cells include cryotherapy, loop diathermy, laser treatment or cold coagulation (organised by gynaecologist).
- Safety net – review if symptoms worsen and arrange follow-up smear tests.
- Information – www.cancerscreening.nhs.uk/cervical.

Role play

Information for doctor	Additional information for role player
Patient: Ms TS *Age*: 28 years *SH*: Single, lives alone, smoker, 15 units alcohol/wk *FH*: Mum has breast cancer. *Information*: Had smear test done 4 weeks ago. Results – moderate dyskaryosis. You are a GP Partner.	*PC*: *"I was asked to come in to discuss my cervical smear results"* *HPC*: Has had intermenstrual and some post-coital bleeding for past few months. No dyspareunia **No abdo pain. No weight loss. LMP 1 week ago. No previous abnormal smear tests. Last smear test 3 years ago. No vaginal discharge.** Has been with current sexual partner for 3 months – having UPSI. *DH*: Microgynon *PMH*: Chlamydia infection 6 months ago. *ICE*: **Worried about why she was called to come in.** Worried that she might have cervical cancer because of the symptoms.

Infertility

- A woman of reproductive age who has not conceived after 1 year of unprotected vaginal sexual intercourse, in the absence of any known cause of infertility, should be offered further clinical assessment and investigation along with her partner (*NICE*, 2013, *CG156*: *Fertility problems*).
- Approximately 1 in 7 couples have difficulty conceiving.

Data gathering

Open question

- *"Can you tell me more about your problems trying to get pregnant?"*

Focused/closed questions

HPC: *"For how long have you been trying to conceive?"*
"When was your last menstrual period?" "Are your periods regular?"
"Have you noticed any bleeding in between your periods or after intercourse?" (red flag)
"Do you have any abdominal pain?"
"How often are you having intercourse?"
"When did you stop using any contraception?"
"Have you ever been pregnant before?" "Any miscarriages or terminations?"
"Has your partner had any children before?"
Take a full sexual history – see *Appendix 2*.

PMH: Any medical conditions? Any history of pelvic inflammatory disease, endometriosis or ectopic pregnancy? Any previous gynaecological surgery? Any history of depression? Any previous STIs? Any history of mumps or testicular problems? ($\male$)

SH: Who lives with you at home? Occupation? Stress? Alcohol/smoking/illicit drug history?

FH: Any family history of fertility problems?

DH: Do you take any regular medications? (teratogenic medications?) Any over the counter medications?

ICE: *"Do you have any thoughts as to why you are having difficulties conceiving?"*

Examination:
- BMI, BP.
- Observe for hirsutism and acne (PCOS).
- Vaginal and speculum examination.
- Abdominal examination.
- In males consider testicular examination.

Clinical management

Investigations
- Blood tests – day 21 progesterone, serum LH and FSH (if irregular menstrual cycle).
- Semen analysis ($\male$).
- Screen for chlamydia before undergoing any uterine instrumentation.
- Rubella screening.
- Pelvic ultrasound scan if indicated from history.

Explanation to patient
- It is important to be reassured that 84% of all couples will conceive within 1 year if they are aged under 40, do not use contraception and have regular intercourse.
- There are various different reasons for fertility problems, some of which are related to the man and some to the woman. Further tests can help to establish the cause.
- There are options to help which include advice about lifestyle changes, medications and referral to a fertility specialist.

Management
(based on *NICE*, 2013, *CG156: Fertility problems*)
- Lifestyle advice – smoking cessation, reduce alcohol and caffeine intake, healthy diet, weight loss, exercise.
- Sexual intercourse every 2–3 days optimises the chance of pregnancy.
- Folic acid supplements.
- Fertility support group.
- Counselling.
- Refer to fertility clinic for further investigations/management if not pregnant after 1 year despite above measures.

- ○ Women with ovulation disorders such as PCOS should be offered clomifene citrate as first line to induce ovulation.
- ○ Couples in which the woman is aged under 40 at the time of treatment, and who have an identifiable cause for their fertility problems, or who have had infertility for at least 2 years duration should be offered up to three stimulated cycles of *in vitro* fertilisation. Unfortunately, due to financial pressures, one in five PCTs have reduced the number of treatment cycles that they are able to offer.

Role play

Information for doctor	Additional information for role player
Patient: Mrs KS *Age*: 32 years *PMH*: Nil *DH*: Nil *Information*: No previous consultations. You are a GP Registrar.	*PC*: *"I've been trying to get pregnant for the past 14 months and have had no success"* *HPC*: **Never been pregnant before.** Partner has never had children. Having unprotected sex 4× weekly. LMP 3 weeks ago. Regular periods. No abdominal pain. No abnormal vaginal bleeding. **No previous STIs.** *SH*: Married 3 years ago. Lives with husband and husband's sister. Accountant. Stressful job. Non-smoker, 5 units alcohol/week. No illicit drug use. *ICE*: **Worried about why she can't conceive and wants referral to fertility specialist.** *O/E*: BMI – 23. BP 110/70. Abdominal and vaginal exam – NAD. No hirsutism or acne.

Menopause

- Permanent cessation of ovarian function, typically occurring around the age of 50 years.
- A woman has reached menopause when she has not had a period for 1 year if over 50 years or if no periods for 2 years in those under 50 years.
- If menopause occurs under the age of 45 years it is known as premature menopause.

Data gathering

Open question

- "Can you tell me more about the menopausal symptoms you have been experiencing?"

Focused/closed questions

HPC: *"When was your last menstrual period?"*

"Have you noticed any changes to your periods?"

"Have you experienced any hot flushes, night sweats or headaches?"
"Have you noticed any mood changes, loss of sex drive or difficulty sleeping?"
"Have you noticed any vaginal dryness?"
"Any abdominal pain or swelling of the abdomen?" (red flag)
"Any bleeding at least 1 year after your periods had stopped?" (red flag)
"Any previous mammograms?" "What were the results?"
"Are you currently using any contraception and if so, what?"

FH: Any family history of premature menopause? Any family history of osteoporosis?

SH: Smoking/alcohol/illicit drug history? Who lives with you at home? Occupation?

ICE: *"Are these symptoms affecting your day to day life?"*

Examination:
- BP, BMI.
- Breast examination.

Clinical management

Investigations
- FSH – helpful in cases of premature menopause.
- Pregnancy test – if relevant.

Explanation to patient
- The menopause naturally occurs when the ovaries stop producing eggs and this results in lower levels of the female hormone oestrogen.
- Various symptoms can occur including mood changes, hot flushes and changes to the vagina and genital skin. For some people these symptoms can be quite debilitating, and treatment is required to help alleviate these symptoms.

Management
(based on *NICE, 2015, NG23: Menopause: diagnosis and management*)
- Lifestyle changes – healthy diet, exercise.
- HRT
  - Usually oestrogen/progesterone combined, or oestrogen only if previous hysterectomy
  - Preparations include tablets, patches and gels
  - Different types include cyclical combined and continuous combined:
    - cyclical combined is suitable for those still experiencing erratic menstrual bleeding. Oestrogen is taken daily, and progesterone is added for the last 12–14 days of the cycle. You will continue to get monthly periods.
    - continuous combined preparations are used once a woman has not had a natural period for at least a year. It involves a daily dose of oestrogen and progesterone and you will not get monthly bleeds.

          ○ Benefits include reducing symptoms of hot flushes and may protect against osteoporosis

          ○ Disadvantages include small increased risk of breast cancer, DVT and endometrial cancer.

- Tibolone – synthetic steroid hormone which helps with hot flushes, sweats and vaginal dryness. Useful for women who cannot take oestrogen and has lower breast cancer risk.
- Clonidine – relieves hot flushes.
- Topical oestrogens.
- Vaginal lubricants
- SSRIs – effective for hot flushes (not licensed).
- Safety net – if no improvement in symptoms return to GP. Patients on HRT should be followed up 3 months after starting treatment, and then 6–12 monthly thereafter. Reviews should include BP, weight and breast examination.

Role play

Information for doctor	Additional information for role player
Patient: Ms PO *Age*: 54 years *SH*: Lives alone, school teacher. Non-smoker. *PMH*: Breast cancer *DH*: Tamoxifen 20 mg OD *Information*: Last saw GP 1 month ago for medication review. You are a locum GP.	*PC*: Menopausal symptoms *HPC*: Experiencing bad hot flushes and some mood swings and vaginal dryness. LMP 8 months ago. No bleeding since. **Also has problems sleeping.** Last mammogram 9 months ago – NAD. *FH*: **Breast cancer (sister).** *ICE*: Would like to know what she could take to help with her menopausal symptoms. *O/E*: BP 120/80, BMI 24. Breast exam – NAD.

Men's health

Haematuria

- Haematuria is the presence of red blood cells in the urine, which can either be macroscopic or microscopic.
- Causes include urinary tract infection, trauma, benign prostatic hyperplasia, TCC of the bladder, renal stones or renal carcinoma.
- Other causes of red urine include certain drugs (e.g. rifampicin) and certain foods (e.g. beetroot).

Data gathering

Open question
- *"Can you tell me more about the blood you noticed in your urine...?"*

Focused/closed questions

HPC: *"When did you first notice blood in your urine?" "Does it happen every time you urinate?"*
"Do you have any pain when you pass urine?" "Have you passed any clots of blood?"
"Any recent bladder surgery?" "Any recent trauma?"
"Any hesitancy when you pass urine?" "Any problems with your urine stream?" "Any urinary incontinence?" "Do you get up at night to pass urine and, if so, how many times?"
"Any weight loss?" (red flag)
"Any associated back pain?" (possible red flag)

PMH: Any previous urology problems? Any past history of kidney stones?

DH: *"Do you take any regular medications?"* Rifampicin? Anticoagulants e.g. warfarin?

SH: Smoking? Occupation? Any exposure to chemicals/dyes?

FH: Any family history of bladder or kidney problems?

ICE: *"Do you have any idea what might be causing the blood in your urine?"*

Examination:
- BP.
- Abdominal examination including palpation of kidneys.
- Rectal examination – to check prostate.

Clinical management

Investigations

- Urine dipstick – check for leucocytes, blood and protein (send for MC&S also).
- Blood test – U&Es and eGFR (to check renal function).
- Consider PSA test if appropriate.
- Urine albumin:creatinine ratio.
- Refer for cystoscopy if no cause found.

Management

- Depends on cause.
- UTI – treat with antibiotics and repeat urine dipstick after treatment.
- Renal tract stone – analgesia and fluids; refer urgently if reduced renal function, pain not controlled or if any signs of obstruction on imaging.
- Urgent referral to urology or nephrology – patients of any age with painless macroscopic haematuria, patients ≥40 years who present with recurrent or persistent UTI associated with haematuria, patients ≥50 years with unexplained microscopic haematuria.

Role play

Information for doctor	Additional information for role player
Patient: Mr SD *Age*: 62 years *SH*: Primary school headteacher. Lives with wife. Non-smoker. Drinks 30 units alcohol/week. *PMH*: Stroke 2010. *DH*: Aspirin 75 mg OD. Simvastatin 40 mg nocte. *Information*: You are a salaried GP. You are seeing this patient today in an emergency appointment.	*PC*: *"This morning I noticed blood in my urine"* *HPC*: First episode this morning. Fresh blood in the toilet pan. **No clots. No dysuria. No trauma. No fever.** No abdominal pain. No weight loss. **No hesitancy but sometimes has poor stream and gets up 3–4 times at night to pass urine.** *ICE*: Worried he might have cancer. *O/E*: BP 140/90. Abdominal exam NAD. PR exam – enlarged smooth prostate.

Benign prostatic hyperplasia

- Benign prostatic hyperplasia (BPH) refers to prostate gland enlargement, which can often cause problems with passing urine.
- Common in older men.
- The figure on the next page shows how you could illustrate the prostate to your patient.

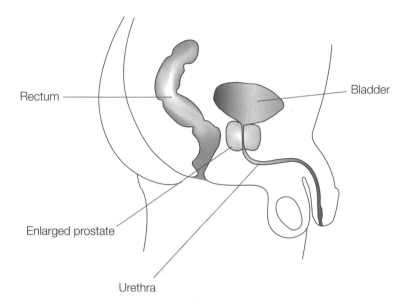

Rectum

Bladder

Enlarged prostate

Urethra

Data gathering

Open question

- *"Do you mind telling me more about your urinary symptoms?"*

Focused/closed questions

HPC: *"Have you been passing urine more frequently than normal? Have you had to rush to get to the toilet to pass urine? Have you had any hesitancy when trying to pass urine, or has the stream of urine been poor?"*

"Do you have any dribbling at the end of the stream of urine? Have you ever been unable to pass urine?" "Have you ever been incontinent of urine?"

"Do you wake up at night to pass urine?" "If so, how many times?"

"Have you noticed any weight loss, bone pains or blood in the urine?" (red flags)

"Any changes in your bowel habit?"

"Any abdominal pain?"

"How many caffeinated drinks do you have each day?"

PMH: Do you suffer with any other medical conditions?

DH: Do you take any regular medications? Diuretics?

SH: Smoking/alcohol/illicit drug history? Occupation?

FH: Any family history of bladder problems?

ICE: *"Do you have any particular worries/concerns about your bladder symptoms?".*

Examination: • Prostate examination (offer chaperone).
   • Abdominal examination – check bladder and kidneys.

Clinical management

Investigations
- Urine dipstick – check for haematuria.
- Blood test – PSA and U&Es. Can check glucose to rule out diabetes.
- Voiding diary.
- Trans-rectal USS prostate.

Explanation to patient
- The prostate gland is found beneath the bladder and is approximately the size of a chestnut. It is only found in men.
- The prostate gland produces fluid which protects and enriches sperm.
- A tube-like structure called the urethra carries urine from the bladder and this runs through the middle of the prostate. The urethra can be narrowed if the prostate enlarges and this is what causes the urinary symptoms.

Management
(based on *NICE*, 2010, *CG97: Lower urinary tract symptoms*)
- Conservative management – watch and wait.
- Double voiding.
- Reduce intake of caffeine and alcohol.
- Bladder training.
- Stop smoking.
- Drug treatment:
    ○ Alpha-blockers, e.g. tamsulosin (relaxes smooth muscle of the prostate).
    ○ 5-alpha reductase inhibitors, e.g. finasteride (blocks the conversion of an enzyme in the prostate that is responsible for prostatic enlargement.
    ○ Anticholinergic, e.g. oxybutynin, to men with symptoms of an overactive bladder.
- Surgery – TURP (transurethral resection of the prostate) or prostatectomy.
- Safety net – if symptoms not improving return to GP.

Role play

Information for doctor	Additional information for role player
Patient: Mr SJ *Age*: 70 years *SH*: Retired, lives alone. Widowed *PMH*: Hypertension *FH*: Nil *DH*: Ramipril 2.5 mg OD *Information*: You are a locum GP in the practice.	*PC*: Urinary problems for the past 4 months. *HPC*: Some terminal dribbling and incomplete emptying. No urgency. Stream generally ok. **No haematuria, weight loss or bone pains. Wakes up 3× at night to pass urine. No dysuria** *ICE*: Worried about prostate cancer as a close friend died from this. *O/E*: Smooth enlarged prostate gland. Abdo exam – NAD.

Prostate cancer

- Cancer which develops from cells in the prostate gland.
- Commonest cancer in men in the UK according to Cancer Research UK (2007, *Prostate cancer – UK incidence statistics*).
- Older men, men with a family history of prostate cancer and men of black African and black Caribbean descent are more at risk.
- Many cases are slow growing and may not affect life expectancy.

Data gathering

Open question

- *"Do you mind telling me more about the problems with your bladder symptoms?"*

Focused/closed questions

HPC: *"Have you been passing urine more frequently than usual? Have you had any difficulties passing urine?"*

"Do you ever have to rush to get to the toilet on time? Do you ever have any dribbling at the end of passing urine or a poor urine stream?"

"Do you wake up at night to pass urine?" " If so, how many times?"

"Have you passed any blood in the urine? (red flag) *Any pain when passing urine? Have you ever been unable to pass urine or not been able to empty your bladder fully?"*

"Do you have any erectile problems?"

"Have you noticed any weight loss or bone pain?" (red flags)

PMH: Do you suffer with any other medical conditions?

DH: Do you take any regular medications?

SH: Smoking/alcohol/drug history? Occupation? Who lives with you at home?

FH: Any family history of prostate cancer or bladder problems?

ICE: *"What do you think might be causing your symptoms?"*

"Do you have any particular worries/concerns about your urinary symptoms?"

Examination:
- Digital rectal examination – to examine prostate.
- Abdominal examination – for palpation of enlarged bladder.

Clinical management

Investigations

- Urine dipstick (check for haematuria and leucocytes).
- PSA test.
- Multiparametric MRI – increasingly offered to some men before biopsy to help with the diagnosis, as well as after biopsy to help with staging.
- Biopsy of the prostate (done by urologist).

Explanation to patient

- Cells in the prostate become abnormal and they multiply 'out of control.'
- Mostly occurs in men over the age of 65 years.
- Risk factors include ageing, family history, ethnicity (commoner in Afro–Caribbean men), diet, and environmental factors.

Management

(based on *NICE, 2014, CG175: Prostate cancer: diagnosis and management*)
- Refer under 2 week wait for suspected cancer if:
  - clinically malignant prostate on digital rectal examination.
  - asymptomatic men with raised or rising age-specific PSA.
  - symptomatic men with high PSA.
  - patients of any age with painless macroscopic haematuria.
  - patients >50 years with unexplained microscopic haematuria.
- Otherwise, consider active surveillance or watchful waiting in low risk men (should offer a PSA test at least annually and always remember to safety net).
- Treatment options for prostate cancer include radical prostatectomy, radiotherapy, chemotherapy, brachytherapy or hormone treatment.
- Patients should be informed that treatment may result in altered physical appearance, change in sexual function and changes in urinary function.

N.B. Screening for prostate cancer is controversial (see *PSA testing* for further information).

Role play

Information for doctor	Additional information for role player
Patient: Mr JE *Age*: 65 years *SH*: Retired, lives with wife. Smokes 10 cigs/day *PMH*: Hypercholesterolaemia *FH*: Nil *DH*: Simvastatin 40 mg nocte *Information*: Saw a GP partner last week due to haematuria, urgency and frequency. Came today for PSA result which is 28 ng/ml. You are a salaried GP.	*PC*: Urinary symptoms. *HPC*: Haematuria, urgency and frequency for the past 6 months. 5 kg weight loss in past 4 months. **No incomplete emptying or terminal dribbling. No bone pain/dysuria/erectile problems.** *ICE*: **Thinks his symptoms are due to 'old age'. Not worried about cancer. Hoping for medication to alleviate his symptoms.** *O/E*: Enlarged craggy prostate. Abdo exam – NAD.

Age Specific PSA

Men <40	<2
Men 40-50	2-2.8
51-60	2.9 - 3.8
61-70	4 - 5.3
>70	5.6 - 7.2

PSA testing

Information for patients
- Blood test that measures the level of prostate specific antigen (PSA) in the blood.
- The PSA is produced by the prostate and is raised in certain conditions, for example: a raised PSA can be a sign of prostate cancer, or BPH, or urinary infection, or a response to a recent examination of the prostate, recent biopsy of the prostate, or the result of exercise.
- PSA naturally rises as men get older and the prostate gland gets bigger.
- Two out of three people with a raised PSA will not have prostate cancer. *2/3 men with ↑PSA don't have cancer.*
- If the PSA result is not raised, it is unlikely to be prostate cancer.
- If the PSA result is mildly elevated, the patient probably doesn't have cancer, but should be monitored.
- If the PSA is very elevated, the patient should be referred to urology following a prostate examination.
- Normal PSA values are generally considered to be <3 ng/ml in those under 60, <4 ng/ml in those aged 60–69 and <5 ng/ml in those over 70.
- Offer patients the following information sheet:
- www.cancerscreening.nhs.uk/prostate/prostate-patient-info-sheet.pdf

Testicular cancer

- Cancer of the testes accounts for just 1% of all male cancers.
- 50% of cases are under 35 years old.
- Risk factors include family history, undescended testes, mumps and possibly environmental factors.
- Curable in 95% of cases.

Data gathering

Open question
- *"Can you tell me more about this testicular lump/swelling that you have noticed?"*

Focused/closed questions
HPC: *"When did you first notice the lump in your testicle?"*
"Is it painful?"
"Has the lump increased in size recently?"
"Do you have any pain or discomfort in the groin?"
"Do you have any urinary symptoms?"
"Have you noticed any weight loss or bone pains?" (red flags)
"Do you have any shortness of breath or are you coughing up any blood?" (red flags)

> *"Do you have any abdominal pain?"*
> *"Any abnormal discharge from the penis?"*

PMH: Any history of undescended testes? Any history of mumps?

FH: Any family history of testicular problems?

SH: Occupation? Smoking/alcohol history?

ICE: *"Was there anything in particular you were concerned about?"*
"How have these symptoms been affecting you?"

Examination:
- Testicular examination (offer chaperone).
- Abdominal examination.
- Examine lymph nodes.

Clinical management

Investigations
- Scrotal ultrasound scan.
- Blood test for tumour markers (AFP, HCG, LDH) – these tests should not delay referral.

Explanation to patient
- The testes are the two male sex organs that sit inside the scrotum.
- They produce sperm and the hormone testosterone which is important in male sexual development.
- The cells that become cancerous are those that are involved in making the sperm.

Management
- Refer to urologist under 2 week rule if suspected testicular cancer (suspicious testicular mass or swelling).
- Surgery and/or chemotherapy/radiotherapy if proven testicular cancer.
- Encourage health promotion – regular testicular examinations.
- Safety net – if symptoms worsen or are not improving return to GP.

Role play

Information for doctor	Additional information for role player
Patient: Mr IK *Age*: 24 years old *SH*: University student, single, lives with 2 friends. Non smoker, no alcohol. *PMH*: Undescended testes. *DH*: Nil *Information*: You are a salaried GP.	*PC*: Testicular swelling *HPC*: Noticed testicular swelling 4 weeks ago. Not worsened since then. Painless swelling. No groin discomfort/pain. **No haematuria. No urinary symptoms. No weight loss.** No abdominal pain. No penile discharge. **Has had MMR.** *FH*: Nil. *ICE*: Unsure what is causing his symptoms. *O/E*: Discrete firm mass palpable in left testis.

Erectile dysfunction

- Erectile dysfunction has been described as the persistent inability to attain and/or maintain an erection sufficient for sexual performance.
- It can have a significant impact on the quality of life of patients and their partners.

Causes to consider

- Blood vessel narrowing secondary to hypertension, smoking, diabetes, or hypercholesterolaemia.
- Psychological causes, e.g. stress, anxiety, depression.
- Medication – e.g. beta-blockers, anti-depressants, cimetidine.
- Neurological causes, e.g. multiple sclerosis, stroke or spinal injury.
- Alcohol and drug abuse.
- Radiotherapy treatment to the pelvis.
- Hormonal causes.

Data gathering

Open question
- *"Can you tell me a bit more about the erectile problems you've been having?"*

Focused/closed questions

HPC: *"How long has the problem been going on for?" "Did it come on quite suddenly?" "Is it getting worse?"*
"Are you ever able to get an erection?" "Do you have difficulty maintaining an erection?" "Do you get early morning erections?"
"How would you describe your sexual desire?
"Do you have any urinary symptoms?" (red flag)
"Have you noticed any blood in your urine?" (red flag)

PMH: Any history of any medical conditions (e.g. prostate cancer, diabetes, hypertension or neurological problems)? *"Any history of depression or previous erectile problems?"*

DH: Any regular medications, e.g. beta-blockers?

SH: Smoking/alcohol/illicit drugs history? Are you in a stable relationship? Any problems with your relationship? Have you had any other sexual partners recently? If so, do you also have erectile problems with this partner? Occupation? Stress? Exercise level?

ICE: *"Do you have any idea what might be causing the erectile problems?"*
"How is this problem affecting you in terms of your relationship?"

Examination: • BMI.
- Blood pressure and heart rate.
- Prostate examination if relevant history.
- External genitalia – check for hypogonadism and Peyronie's disease.

Clinical management

Investigations

- Blood tests:
  - fasting glucose and cholesterol, U&Es, PSA.
  - serum testosterone, FSH, LH and prolactin.
  - TFTs, LFTs if clinically indicated.

Explanation to patient

- Erectile dysfunction is usually caused by poor blood flow to the penis.
- The commonest reason for this is narrowing of the blood vessels due to formation of fatty plaques called atheromas.
- Psychological reasons are other common causes of erectile dysfunction.
- Smoking and alcohol are common risk factors.
- Various different medical conditions and medications can also predispose to erectile problems, for example diabetes, high blood pressure, beta-blockers and anti-depressant medications.

Management

- Lifestyle advice (smoking cessation, healthy diet, exercise).
- If possible psychiatric cause, consider counselling, reducing stress levels and/or anti-depressants.
- If related to medication consider stopping the medication or changing to an alternative.
- Medication – PDE5 inhibitors, e.g. sildenafil, tadalafil (work by increasing blood flow to the penis); these are only available on a private script unless the patient has a specific medical condition which qualifies for NHS prescription (see www.bnf.org). Herbal remedies – ginseng or yohimbine.
- Injection therapy, vacuum devices, penile prosthesis.
- Alprostadil cream (Vitaros) – new option to consider.
- Patient information leaflet – www.patient.co.uk/health/Erectile-Dysfunction-(Impotence).htm.
- Safety net – if not improving after 4–6 weeks return to GP.

Role play

Information for doctor	Additional information for role player
Patient: Mr DG *Age*: 48 years old *SH*: Accountant, married with 2 children. *DH*: Nil *PMH*: Nil *FH*: Diabetes *Information*: You are a GP Registrar. This patient has never been seen in the surgery before.	*PC*: Erectile problems. *HPC*: Four month history of difficulty getting and maintaining erection. **Gets early morning erections. Marriage problems for past 6 months.** Feels low in mood. Poor sleep. Stress at work. **Low libido. No urinary symptoms.** *ICE*: **Very worried that these erectile problems are exacerbating the problems with his marriage.** Keen to have Viagra to improve things. *O/E*: BMI 24, BP 120/80. PR exam – NAD.

Testicular conditions

- Possible testicular conditions include hydrocoele, varicocoele and epididymo-orchitis.

Hydrocoele
- Collection of fluid in the scrotal sac around the testes.
- Usually unilateral but can be bilateral.
- Normally painless.
- Trans-illuminates on examination.

Varicocoele
- Collection of dilated veins in the scrotum due to a problem with the valves.
- Similar to varicose veins in the legs.
- Usually causes no symptoms but can cause discomfort.
- Affects 1 in 7 men.
- Associated with a small increased risk of infertility.

Epididymo-orchitis
- Inflammation of the epididymis and/or testis.
- Commonly caused by an infection (UTI or STI).
- Treatment is usually with antibiotics.

Data gathering

Open question
- *"Can you tell me more about your symptoms?"*

Focused/closed questions
HPC: *"Do you have any pain when passing urine?" "Any scrotal swelling?" "Any tenderness around the scrotum?" "Any discharge from your penis?" "Have you noticed any blood in your urine?" "Any weight loss?" "Have you noticed any lumps in your testes or have you experienced any pain in your testes?"* (red flags)
Take a sexual history – see *Appendix 2*.

PMH: Any history of testicular problems or sexually transmitted infections?

FH Any family history of testicular problems?

SH Smoking/alcohol/illicit drug use? Occupation?

ICE: *"Do you have any thoughts as to what might be causing your symptoms?" "What were you hoping we might be able to do to help?"*

Examination:
- Temperature.
- Testicular examination (including trans-illumination with pen torch) and examination of penis.
- Examination of lymph nodes.

Clinical management

Investigations
- Scrotal ultrasound scan.
- Urine dipstick and/or MC&S
- STI screening – urethral swab and urine sample.

Management
- Hydrocoele – can leave alone or offer surgery/drainage.
- Varicocoele – can leave alone, or offer surgery to tie off enlarged veins or injection therapy to block affected veins.
- Epididymo-orchitis – antibiotics and/or analgesia. See www.bashh.org/guidelines for further information.
- Safety net – if symptoms not improving to review again. If any signs suggestive of testicular torsion (severe testicular pain) refer immediately.

Role play

Information for doctor	Additional information for role player
Patient: Mr AJ *Age*: 28 years old *SH*: Unemployed, lives alone, single *PMH*: Nil *DH*: Nil *Information*: You are a GP partner and have never seen this patient before.	*PC*: Painful scrotum. *HPC*: 1 week history of scrotal pain. Urethral discharge. **Dysuria. No urgency or frequency. No testicular swelling or masses. Had unprotected sexual intercourse with casual female partner 2 weeks ago.** Not ever had STI check. *ICE*: Worried about an STI. *O/E*: Apyrexial. Tenderness and swelling of epididymis.

Vasectomy

- Male sterilisation.
- Permanent form of contraception.
- Available on NHS but reversal is usually not.

Data gathering

Open question
- *"Can you tell me a bit more about why you would like a vasectomy?"*

Focused/closed questions
HPC: *"Are you currently in a relationship?" "If so, how old is your partner?" "Have you had children in the past?" "If so, how many?" "Are these with the same partner?"*

> *"What are you currently using for contraception?"*
> *"Have you discussed the vasectomy with your partner?" "How does she feel?" "Have you considered alternative options?"*

PMH: Any medical conditions or previous surgery?

SH: Who lives with you at home? Occupation?

ICE: *"Do you know what a vasectomy entails?"*

Examination:
- BMI.
- Blood pressure.

Clinical management

Explanation to patient

- Small operation to cut the vas deferens (the tube that takes sperm from the testes to the penis).
- If the vas deferens is cut, the sperm are unable to get into the semen that is ejaculated during sex.
- It can usually be done under local anaesthetic.
- The failure rate is about 1 in 2000.
- You may experience some tenderness and bruising afterwards, but a vasectomy has no effect on sex drive. Most patients are back to work within a few days and return to normal function within 2 weeks.
- Approximately 8 weeks after the operation you will need to produce two semen samples approx 3–6 weeks apart to ensure that these samples are clear of sperm. You should use contraception with your partner until these semen samples are clear of sperm.
- Offer information leaflet www.nhs.uk/conditions/contraception-guide/pages/vasectomy-male-sterilisation.aspx.

Management

- Refer to a urologist for a vasectomy.
- Safety net – GP to review if any further concerns or complications post-operatively.

Role play

Information for doctor	Additional information for role player
Patient: Mr JR Age: 40 years old SH: Solicitor. Lives with wife, has 3 children. PMH: IDDM DH: Novorapid 18 units TDS, Lantus 30 units OD. Information: You are a locum GP. This patient came to see the nurse last week for a routine diabetic check. He mentioned that he wanted a vasectomy.	PC: **Has 3 children all with the same partner (aged 42 years).** Has discussed with his wife and they both don't want any more children. **They have been using condoms for contraception.** ICE: Wants a permanent method of contraception as doesn't want any more children.

Sexual health

Chlamydia

- Most common sexually transmitted infection in the UK.
- The highest prevalence rates are in 15–24 year olds.
- Causes no symptoms in around 70% of females and 50% of males.
- Caused by the bacterium *Chlamydia trachomatis.*

Data gathering

Open question
- *"Can you tell me more about the symptoms you have been experiencing?"*

Focused/closed questions

HPC: Any vaginal discharge (♀) / urethral discharge (♂)? *"If so, when did it start?" "What colour/consistency is it?" "Does it smell?"*
Any abdominal pain? (red flag)
Any burning pain when you pass urine / vaginal bleeding (♀) / penile pain (♂)?
"Any vaginal bleeding in between periods or any bleeding after sex?" (red flags)
"Any pain during intercourse?"
"Any vaginal itching or sores?"
Take sexual history – see *Appendix 2.*

SH: Who lives with you at home? Smoking/alcohol/illicit drug history? Are you currently in a relationship?

ICE: *"Do you have any thoughts as to what might be causing these symptoms?"*
"What concerns do you have about these symptoms?"

Examination:
- Abdominal examination.
- Speculum and vaginal examination (♀).
- External genitalia examination including inguinal lymph nodes (♂).

Clinical management
(based on *BASHH*, 2015, *UK National guideline for the management of infection with* Chlamydia trachomatis)

Investigations
- Females: If symptomatic take vulvo-vaginal or endocervical swabs for chlamydia and gonorrhoea NAAT testing. If asymptomatic offer a low vaginal self swab. Also perform a vaginal swab for candida and bacterial vaginosis.

- Males: First catch urine sample for chlamydia and gonorrhoea NAAT testing. Also do rectal swabs for men who have sex with men.
- Screening for other STIs – e.g. blood test for HIV and syphilis.

Explanation to patient

- Chlamydia infection in women usually affects the cervix and/or womb. In men, it affects the urethra (tube) in the penis.
- If you are infected with chlamydia it is essential that you take treatment even if you do not have any symptoms, because the infection may spread and cause serious complications and you can also still pass on the infection to your sexual partner(s).
- Condoms are the only effective means of preventing STIs except for abstinence.

Management

- Antibiotics – e.g. azithromycin 1 g stat or doxycycline 100 mg BD for 7 days (avoid all sex for 7 days after treatment of both patient and partner).
- Contact tracing.
- Pregnancy test (♀). If pregnant should test for cure after treatment.
- Offer details of local sexual health clinic for more detailed screening.
- Patient education and information leaflet.
- Offer annual screening for all sexually active people under the age of 25 years.
- Safety net – if symptoms don't resolve to return to GP.

Role play

Information for doctor		Additional information for role player
Patient:	Ms JJ	PC: "I've had some vaginal discharge for the past few days"
Age:	19 years	HPC: Had unprotected sexual intercourse 10 days ago with casual partner. **LMP 3 weeks ago. No irregular menstrual bleeding. Thin clear coloured discharge. Not smelly. No dysuria. No abdominal pain.**
SH:	College student. Lives with parents.	
PMH:	Nil	Sexual history: Vaginal sex only with male partner from UK. Not using any contraceptive.
DH:	Nil	ICE: **Worried she may have got chlamydia as the guy she had sex with told her after that he had chlamydia.**
Information:	Was seen by GP Partner 8 months ago and was treated for chlamydia infection.	O/E: Thin greyish discharge seen on speculum examination.

Pelvic inflammatory disease

- PID is an infection of the female upper genital tract (uterus, fallopian tubes and/or ovaries).
- Most cases are due to ascending infection from the cervix or vagina.
- Commonest infective causes are chlamydia or gonorrhoea.
- Most commonly occurs in the 15–25 year age group.

Data gathering

Open question
- *"Can you tell me more about the symptoms you have been experiencing?"*

Focused/closed questions

HPC: *"Have you been experiencing any abdominal pain?"* *"Where exactly is the pain?"* *"Does the pain radiate?"* *"When did the pain first start?"*
"Do you get any pain during intercourse?"
"Do you notice any bleeding after sex or between periods?" (red flags)
"Do you have any pain when passing urine?"
Any vaginal discharge? Fever?
"When was your last menstrual period?" (always consider ectopic pregnancy)
Take sexual history – see *Appendix 2*

PMH: Any previous sexually transmitted infections?
Any previous pelvic surgery?

SH: Smoking/alcohol/illicit drug history? Who lives with you at home? Occupation?

ICE: *"How have these symptoms been generally affecting you?"*

Examination:
- Check temperature – may have fever >38°C.
- Abdominal examination.
- Vaginal examination – check for cervical motion tenderness and adnexal tenderness.
- Speculum examination.

Clinical management

Investigations
- Endocervical or vaginal swabs for gonorrhoea and chlamydia NAATs.
- Vaginal swab for other infections.
- Blood test – WCC, CRP.
- Pregnancy test.
- Pelvic ultrasound scan and/or laparoscopy – if recommended by a specialist.

Explanation to patient

- Pelvic inflammatory disease is usually caused by an infection in the womb or around the ovaries which has spread up from the vaginal area.
- It usually causes abdominal pain.
- Antibiotics are usually enough to treat the infection and improve symptoms.
- It is important that it is treated early as it can affect your fertility if symptoms go untreated for a long time. In pregnancy, one complication may be an ectopic pregnancy where the fetus grows outside of the womb.

Management

(based on *BASHH*, 2011, *UK national guideline for the management of pelvic inflammatory disease*)

- Have a low threshold for empirical treatment of PID with a broad-spectrum antibiotic.
- Mild–moderate PID – oral ofloxacin 400 mg twice daily plus oral metronidazole 400 mg twice daily for 14 days.
- If severe symptoms, admit to hospital for IV antibiotics and/or consideration for surgery (salpingectomy). Consider appropriate analgesia before transfer to hospital.
- Also admit to hospital if a surgical emergency cannot be excluded, for PID in pregnancy, tubo-ovarian abscess, or for poor response to oral treatment.
- Offer contact tracing if chlamydia or gonorrhoea are confirmed.
- Safety net – follow up in 72 hours or sooner if necessary and again after treatment is completed.

Role play

Information for doctor	Additional information for role player
Patient: Ms SR *Age*: 21 years *SH*: University student *PMH*: Nil *DH*: Nil *Information*: You are a GP Registrar and SR is a temporary patient.	*PC:* Abdominal pain *HPC:* Pain in lower abdomen intermittently for the past month. No radiation. Pain during intercourse also. **No IMB/PCB. Has some vaginal discharge – clear thin discharge, no odour.** No dysuria. **LMP 2 weeks ago.** *Sexual history:* **Has had about 10 different sexual partners in the past 6 months.** Last had sex 1 week ago (unprotected sexual intercourse). *ICE:* Worried about STIs as has never been tested. *O/E*: Afebrile. Tenderness in left iliac fossa. Abdomen soft. Mild left adnexal tenderness. Cervical motion tenderness.

Emergency contraception

- Contraception which is taken after unprotected intercourse to protect against pregnancy.
- The three main types are Levonelle and ulipristal pills and the IUCD.

Data gathering

Open question
- *"Why are you requesting emergency contraception today?"*

Focused/closed questions

HPC: *"When did you have unprotected intercourse?"*

"Did you consent to intercourse?"

"Have there been any other episodes of unprotected intercourse since your last period?"

"When was your last menstrual period?"

"Any abdominal pain?" (red flag)

"Any vaginal bleeding since your last period?"

"Have you used emergency contraception before?"

"What contraception do you usually use?" "Why did it fail?"

PMH: Any past medical problems? Any previous pregnancies? Any previous STIs?

SH: Smoking/alcohol/illicit drug history? Relationship? Who lives with you at home? Support? Occupation?

ICE: *"Do you know how emergency contraception works?"*

Examination
- BP and weight.
- Abdominal examination – if there is abdominal pain.

Clinical management

Investigations
- Pregnancy test – if appropriate from the history.

Explanation to patient
- Emergency contraception is used to prevent you getting pregnant if you have unprotected sex.
- There are two main types – the emergency contraceptive pill or an intra-uterine contraceptive device (IUCD) which can be inserted into the womb up to five days after having unprotected sex.
- The pill is the most commonly used emergency contraception. The progesterone pill is called Levonelle, and this is taken as a one-off dose as soon as possible after unprotected sex. It either prevents or delays the release of an egg or prevents the

fertilised egg from implanting in the womb. If used within 24 hours of unprotected intercourse it is about 95% effective. If used within 48 hours it is 85% effective, and if used within 72 hours it is about 58% effective. If a patient vomits within 2 hours they should take another pill as soon as possible.

- The other emergency contraceptive pill, ulipristal, was found to be 97% effective if used within 72 hours in a recent study (*Faculty of Sexual and Reproductive Healthcare*, 2009, *New product review October*). Ulipristal can be used up to 5 days after UPSI.
- The IUCD (copper coil) can be used for emergency contraception (it is the most effective option) and then for on-going contraception.
- After using emergency contraception it is important to use barrier contraception if having sexual intercourse before your next period. Also consider and discuss long term contraceptive options.
- If after using emergency contraception your next period is late, it is important that you do a pregnancy test and see your GP as soon as possible.

Management
- Levonelle or ulipristal.
- IUCD.
- Contraception advice and education.
- Sexual health promotion.
- Give patient information leaflet – www.fpa.org.uk.
- Safety net – if next period is delayed or very light come back to see GP.

Role play

Information for doctor	Additional information for role player
Patient: Ms LJ *Age*: 15 years *SH*: School pupil, smokes 10 cigs/day *PMH*: Asthma *DH*: Salbutamol 1–2 puffs PRN, beclomethasone 1–2 puffs BD.	*PC*: "*I had unprotected sex 2 days ago and would like the morning after pill*" *HPC*: **Had unprotected sexual intercourse with casual partner 48 hours ago.** Not on any regular contraception. No other episodes of UPSI since last period. No abdominal pain. No previous pregnancies. **Never had STI check before. LMP 3 weeks ago.** *ICE*: Worried about getting pregnant. Keen to try the implant for long term contraception. Wants emergency pill today and not keen on IUCD.

Combined oral contraceptive pill

- Contains two hormones, progesterone and oestrogen.
- Works by preventing ovulation, thickening cervical mucus to prevent fertilisation and thinning the lining of the uterus to prevent implantation.

- It is over 99% effective if used correctly.
- In England, Wales and Northern Ireland it is lawful to provide contraceptive advice and treatment to young people without parental consent, provided that the practitioner is satisfied that the Fraser criteria for competence are met:
  - The young person understands the practitioner's advice.
  - The young person cannot be persuaded to inform their parents, or will not allow the practitioner to inform the parents, that contraceptive advice has been sought.
  - The young person is likely to begin or to continue having intercourse with or without contraceptive treatment.
  - Unless she receives contraceptive advice or treatment, the young person's physical or mental health (or both) are likely to suffer.
- In Scotland, although the Fraser Guidelines are sometimes used by health professionals, they have no authority in Scottish law. The only criterion when determining 'competency' is that the child understands the nature and consequence of the treatment.

Data gathering

Open question
- *"Why would you like to start taking the combined contraceptive pill?"*
- *"Have you considered any of the longer-acting forms of contraception, as they don't depend on you remembering to take them?"*

Focused/closed questions
HPC: *"When was your last menstrual period?"*
"Are your periods regular?"
"Are you currently using any form of contraception?"
"Do you suffer with heavy periods?"
"Do you ever suffer from migraines?" "If so, do you experience any warning signs beforehand, e.g. flashing lights?" (red flag)

PMH: Any history of high blood pressure, heart disease, liver disease, breast cancer or DVT? (red flags)

FH: Any family history of breast cancer, DVT, stroke or heart disease?

DH: Do you take any regular medications? St John's Wort? Enzyme inducers, e.g. carbamazepine, rifampicin?

SH: Do you smoke?

ICE: *"What do you know about the pill?"*

Examination:
- BP.
- BMI.

Clinical management

Investigations
- Nil

Explanation to patient

- The most common type of pill is the 21 day pill, in which each month you take one tablet a day for 21 days and then no tablets for 7 days. During the 7 day break you will expect to get a 'withdrawal' bleed.
- If you start the pill on the first day of your period, or up to day 5 of a regular 28 day cycle, you will be protected from pregnancy straight away. If you start the pill at any other time, you will need to use additional contraception for the first 7 days after starting the pill.
- The advantages of the combined pill are, it usually makes your bleeds regular, lighter and less painful. It may also help with premenstrual symptoms, and it may reduce the risk of cancer of the ovary, uterus and colon. It may also protect against pelvic inflammatory disease.
- The disadvantages are that you may experience side effects, such as headaches, nausea, breast tenderness and mood changes. The pill may also increase your blood pressure, and it does not protect against sexually transmitted infections. There is also a slight increased risk of developing a DVT. Research suggests that there may be a very small increased risk of developing breast cancer or cervical cancer with longer use of hormonal contraception.
- Possible side effects include breast tenderness, bloating, and mood changes.
- Missing one pill anywhere in the pack, or starting the pill one day late is not a problem. If you have missed more than one pill, refer to the missed pill rules (www.fpa.org.uk).
- If you have diarrhoea the pill may be less effective and extra precautions may be needed.

Management

- Initial 3 month check followed by 6 monthly pill check (including BP check).
- Patient education, including an information leaflet and explanation of the missed pill rules.

Role play

Information for doctor	Additional information for role player
Patient: Ms JE *Age*: 15 years *SH*: Lives with parents. School pupil. Non-smoker *FH*: Nil *PMH*: Nil *Information*: You are a GP registrar.	*PC*: "*I would like to start on the pill*" *HPC*: Has a new boyfriend and they have started being sexually active. **Consensual sex. Doesn't want to inform her parents but will continue to have sex anyway. Using condoms currently. LMP 3 weeks ago. Periods regular. No history of DVT/breast cancer/heart disease/migraine.** *ICE*: Wants to try the pill as some of her friends at school take it. *O/E*: BP 120/80, BMI 23.

Termination of pregnancy

- One-fifth of all pregnancies are terminated worldwide.
- 90% of all abortions are carried out at under 13 weeks of gestation.
- The 1967 Abortion Act allows termination before 24 weeks of gestation if:
  - it reduces the risk to a woman's life, or
  - it reduces the risk to her physical or mental health, or
  - it reduces the risk to the physical or mental health of her existing children, or
  - the baby is at substantial risk of being seriously mentally or physically handicapped.
- There is no upper limit on gestational time if there is a risk to the mother's life or risk of grave permanent injury to the mother's physical/mental health or if there is substantial risk that, if the child were born, it would suffer such physical or mental abnormalities as to be seriously handicapped.

Data gathering

Open question
- *"Why do you want to have a termination?"*

Focused/closed questions
HPC: *"How did you find out you were pregnant?"*
"When was your last menstrual period?"
"Have you ever been pregnant before?"
"Were you using any contraception?" "If so, what?"
"Was this with a regular partner?"
"Did you consent to sex?"
"Have you spoken to anyone else about this?"
"Have you got any abdominal pain or fever?" (red flags)
"Have you thought about other options, for example adoption?"

PMH: *"Have you had any previous terminations?"*
"Have you had any previous pelvic surgery?"
Any history of depression?

SH: *"Are you currently in a relationship?" "Have you discussed this with your partner?"*
Who lives with you at home? Support network? *"Have you ever been a victim of domestic violence?"* (see *Appendix 7*)
Occupation?

ICE: *"Do you have any ideas about what a termination entails?"*
"Do you have any concerns about having a termination?"

Examination:
- BP, BMI.
- Abdominal examination.

Clinical management

Investigations

- Pregnancy test.
- Chlamydia screening and rhesus status will be checked if she chooses a termination.
- Ultrasound scan – dating and viability scan is undertaken in some cases prior to the TOP.

Explanation to patient

- There are different types of termination depending on how many weeks pregnant you are:
  - Medical termination (up to 9 weeks pregnant) – you attend a hospital/clinic twice, on two separate days. You are given two medications 48 hours apart (mifepristone and prostaglandin). Mifepristone blocks the hormones that help a pregnancy to continue. Prostaglandins make your womb contract and cause vaginal bleeding and cramping to expel the products of the pregnancy.
  - Vacuum aspiration is used for pregnancies between 7 and 15 weeks of pregnancy. A tube is inserted into your womb through the cervix and suction is applied to remove the womb contents.
  - Dilation and evacuation (D&E) is used for pregnancies over 15 weeks. It is a surgical procedure whereby the neck of the womb is dilated and the womb is evacuated of its contents.

Management

- Counsel the patient to ensure she is comfortable with her decision and discuss other options.
- Refer for termination of pregnancy, e.g. Marie Stopes Clinic (note that as a doctor, it is your legal right to refuse to certify a woman for an abortion if you have a moral objection, although you should refer immediately to another doctor who is willing to certify the patient).
- Arrange follow-up which should include a discussion about contraception and counselling if required.
- Safety net – see GP or go straight to A&E if fever or abdominal pain or heavy vaginal bleeding.

Role play

Information for doctor	Additional information for role player
Patient: Ms AL *Age*: 25 years *SH*: Waitress, lives with boyfriend *FH*: Nil *PMH*: Nil *DH*: Nil *Information*: Newly registered patient. You are a locum GP.	*PC*: "'I've just found out that I'm pregnant and I would like to have a termination". *HPC*: LMP 7 weeks ago. **No previous pregnancies.** Was using condoms but sometimes forgot. Hasn't discussed with boyfriend. Doesn't want to tell him. Not keen on alternative options. No abdominal pain or fever. *SH*: **Has a supportive friend she can talk to.** *ICE*: **Doesn't feel ready to have children yet. Not financially stable. Having relationship problems also.** *O/E*: BP 100/70, BMI 20.

Care and palliative care of people with cancer

Palliative care and pain management

- GPs will often be the first point of contact for palliative care patients in the community.
- Common problems encountered in palliative care include inadequate pain control, vomiting, constipation and depression.
- It is important that the patient feels well supported in the community, and GPs should work alongside the community palliative care team, to offer ongoing help and support to the patient and their families.
- Following the demise of the Liverpool Care Pathway, NICE published its *Care of Dying Adults* guideline, *NG31*, in December 2015.

Data gathering

Open question
- *"Can you tell me what problems you have been experiencing?"*

Focused/closed questions

HPC: *"Are you currently experiencing any pain?" "If so, where is the pain?"*
"What type of pain is it?" "How severe is the pain?"
"Are you experiencing any nausea or vomiting, or any constipation?"
"Are you passing urine OK?"
"Any breathlessness?" (red flag)
"How is your appetite?"
"How is your mood?"
"Are you sleeping OK?"

DH: *"What medications are you currently taking?"*

SH: Who is living with you at home? Support network? How are you coping? Carers? Finances?

ICE: *"How were you hoping we could help you today?"*
"Do you have any particular worries or concerns about your illness?"

Examination: • Specific to symptoms, e.g. abdominal, respiratory, etc.

Clinical management

Investigations

- If abdominal pain, consider abdominal X-ray.
- If SOB, consider CXR.

Explanation to patient

- Palliative care aims to provide relief from pain and other distressing symptoms, and also offers a support system to help you as the patient, and your loved ones through this difficult time.

Management

Pain management

- Use a pain assessment tool to adequately assess the pain before starting or changing analgesics.
- If pain control is required use the analgesic ladder and regularly review:
  - Step 1 (Mild pain) – use paracetamol +/- NSAIDs.
  - Step 2 (Moderate pain) – use weak opioids such as codeine, dihydrocodeine or tramadol.
  - Step 3 (Moderate–severe pain) – use strong opioids. Morphine is the drug of first choice. Start with 5–10 mg 4 hourly (use lower doses in the elderly or those with renal impairment). Increase in 30–50% increments to achieve pain control.
  - If the morphine dose exceeds 300 mg in 24 hours seek specialist advice.
  - When prescribing opiates also prescribe laxatives and if required, an anti-emetic.
  - For maintenance treatment, you can continue with 4-hourly immediate release morphine or change to 12-hourly modified release morphine.
  - Consider fentanyl or buprenorphine patches if oral opioids unsuitable.

Symptom control

(based on *NICE*, 2015, *NG31: Care of dying adults* guideline)

- Nausea and vomiting – seek and treat any reversible causes (e.g. medications, infection, constipation, hypercalcaemia). Treatments include metoclopramide, domperidone and cyclizine.
- Breathlessness – treat any reversible causes (e.g. infection, effusion, PE*). Treatment options include handheld fan, relaxation and breathing exercises, low dose opioids and bronchodilators. Supplemental oxygen is not recommended unless significant hypoxaemia.
  *requires hospital treatment.
- Constipation – clarify cause before starting treatment, e.g. opioids, dehydration, immobility, hypercalcaemia. Encourage good fluid intake. Can try senna, lactulose, Movicol or co-danthramer in terminally ill patients.
- Bone pain – opiates, NSAIDS and/or radiotherapy.
- Delirium – causes include opioid or sedative drugs, drug withdrawal, dehydration, urinary retention or electrolyte disturbance. Treat any underlying causes. First line drug is haloperidol 0.5–3 mg PO or SC daily. Second choice is benzodiazepines,

e.g. lorazepam 0.5–1 mg PO or SL. Nurse in quiet area with minimal noise and adequate lighting.

- Emergencies:
  - Haemorrhage – give sedation if distressed and/or dying patient. Consider emergency referral.
  - Hypercalcaemia – hydration and bisphosphonates.
  - Seizures – prophylactic anticonvulsant if structural cause. Midazolam or rectal diazepam if dying patient.
  - Spinal cord compression – emergency referral to A&E.
- Last days of life – care should be reviewed on at least a daily basis, and an individualized care plan should be in place. Gather and document the person's wishes and the views of those important to them. Avoid unnecessary investigation unless there is a clear clinical indication which may improve quality of care. Hydration status should be carefully assessed and patients offered hydration if appropriate, in line with their wishes. Anticipatory prescribing is recommended for the key symptoms of pain, breathlessness, anxiety and agitation, nausea and vomiting and noisy respiratory secretions.

Role play

Information for doctor	Additional information for role player
Patient: Mrs JC *Age*: 47 years *SH*: Married with 2 children. Currently receiving disability living allowance. *PMH*: Metastatic breast cancer (known lung mets) *DH*: MST 30 mg BD, oramorph 5 ml PRN, lactulose 10 ml BD. *Information*: Booked emergency appointment today. You are a salaried GP.	*PC*: "*I have a lot of back pain and am having difficulty getting out of the house now*". *HPC*: Worsening back pain for the past couple of days. Pain over vertebrae. No radiation. Has to walk with a stick. Is already taking high doses of analgesia. Bowels last opened 2 days ago. No nausea or vomiting. Passing urine OK. No leg numbness. *ICE*: Would like some stronger pain relief. *O/E*: Cachectic. Tenderness over lower lumbar vertebrae.

Mental health

Anxiety

- Generalised anxiety disorder is a condition where you have excessive anxiety on most days.
- The cause is unknown, although it may be triggered by a stressful event or there may be a genetic component.
- Treatment includes CBT, medication or self help.

Data gathering

Open questions

- *"Can you tell me more about the anxiety you have been experiencing?"*
- *"What do you mean when you say you are anxious?"*

Focused/closed questions

HPC: *"How long have you experienced these feelings for?"*

       "How frequently do these symptoms occur?"

       "Are there any particular triggers?"

       "Do you ever have an awareness of your heart beating quickly?"

       Any SOB/dry mouth/nausea?

       "Do you ever experience episodes of feeling irritable?"

       "Do you have problems sleeping?"

       "Do you ever avoid certain situations due to fear or anxiety?"

       "Have you ever had any thoughts of harming yourself or suicide?" (red flags)

PMH: *"Have you ever had any anxiety or panic attacks in the past?"*

       Any past history of depression or psychiatric illness?

DH: Are you on any regular medications?

FH: *"Are you aware of any family history of mental illness or anxiety?"*

SH: Who lives with you at home? Support network? Occupation? Smoking/alcohol/illicit drug history? Daily caffeine intake?

ICE: *"How is this problem affecting your day to day life?"*

Examination: Blood pressure, pulse.

- Cardiac examination – if relevant.
- Mental state examination.

Clinical management

Investigations
- ECG.
- Blood test – consider TFTs and glucose.

Explanation to patient
- Anxiety is the unpleasant feeling you get when you feel worried, uneasy or distressed about something that may or may not be about to happen.
- It can result in physical symptoms such as nausea, dry mouth, rapid breathing and fast heart rate.
- Feeling anxious is sometimes perfectly normal. However, people with generalised anxiety disorder find it hard to control their worries. Their feelings of anxiety are more constant and often affect their daily life.

Management
(based on *NICE, 2007, CG22: Anxiety*)
- Self help strategies.
- Exercise.
- Cognitive behavioural therapy.
- Medication – SSRI for minimum of 6 months or propranolol for short term use. Benzodiazepines can be used, but not for longer than 2–4 weeks.
- Offer information about support groups.
- If no improvement despite the above measures, refer to psychiatry.
- Safety net – arrange follow-up appointment to monitor progress.

Role play

Information for doctor		Additional information for role player
Patient:	Mr SW	*PC*: Feeling very anxious for the past month. Has had panic attacks whilst on the train going to work.
Age:	43 years	
SH:	Single, works as an investment banker, smoker, drinks 40 units alcohol/wk. Drinks 3–4 cups of coffee daily.	*HPC*: Difficulty concentrating, **poor sleep**. Has a very stressful job. **Worried about redundancy.** Generally low mood. Gets dry mouth and palpitations during panic attacks. Also hyperventilates. **No suicidal ideation.**
PMH:	Depression	
DH:	Fluoxetine 40 mg OD	
FH:	Brother has depression.	
Information:	You are a GP Partner. You last saw this patient 1 month ago for a medication review.	*ICE*: **Would like some medication to help with his anxiety.**
		O/E: HR 90 bpm, regular; BP 130/80; cardiac exam – NAD. Mental state examination – appears very anxious.

Depression

- Describes a state of persistent low mood, severe enough to interfere with everyday life.
- It affects 1 in 5 people at some point in their lives.
- Symptoms include low mood, loss of interest and enjoyment, low energy, feelings of guilt and worthlessness, and changes in appetite and sleep pattern.
- Management includes watchful waiting, self help, talking therapies and anti-depressants.

Data gathering

Open question
- *"Can you tell me about your low mood?"*

Focused/closed questions
HPC: *"Over the past month have you felt down, depressed or hopeless?"*
"When did you first start feeling low in mood?"
"Did anything trigger it off?"
How is your sleep/concentration/self esteem?
"How would you describe your energy levels?"
"How has your appetite been?"
"Have you had little interest or pleasure in doing things?"
How are you functioning at work/college/school?
"Have you ever felt so low that you felt like you didn't want to carry on with life?" (red flag) *"If so, had you made any plans?"* *"What stopped you from following through with these plans?"*

PMH: Any previous problems with depression/mental illness? Any past psychiatric admissions? Any previous suicide/self harm attempts? (red flag)

DH: Are you on any regular medications? (beware of the potentially disinhibiting effects of benzodiazepines in someone depressed and suicidal)

FH: Any family history of depression?

SH: Who lives with you at home? Support network? Occupation? Smoking/alcohol/illicit drug history?

Examination: • Mental state examination (see *Appendix 3*).

Clinical management

Investigations
- PHQ-9 questionnaire.
- Bloods – e.g. FBC, TFTs and calcium to rule out other possible causes.

Explanation to patient

- The word 'depression' is used to describe everyday feelings of low mood which can affect us all from time to time. Feeling sad or fed up is a normal reaction to experiences that are upsetting, stressful or difficult; those feelings will usually pass.
- If you are affected by depression, you are not 'just' sad or upset. You have an illness which means that intense feelings of persistent sadness, helplessness and hopelessness are accompanied by physical effects such as sleeplessness and loss of energy.

Management

(based on *NICE*, 2009, *CG90: Depression in adults (update)*)

- Conservative – exercise, diet, sleep hygiene.
- If mild depression, consider watchful waiting or recommend a guided self help programme based on CBT.
- In mild to moderate depression, consider short term psychological treatment (e.g. CBT or counselling).
- In severe depression consider combination treatment of an anti-depressant* (SSRI) and individual CBT.
- If immediate risk to self or others, consider an urgent referral to the mental health services.
- Safety net – always arrange follow-up and ask the patient to return sooner if their depressive symptoms worsen.

*Anti-depressants: consider if moderate/severe depression or mild depression unresponsive to initial treatments. Review 2 weeks after starting, or sooner if high suicide risk. Consider increasing dose or changing drug if no improvement after 3–4 weeks. Continue for 6 months after remission.

Role play

Information for doctor	Additional information for role player
Patient: Mr HA *Age*: 34 years *SH*: Unemployed. Lives alone. Wife in Pakistan with his children. *FH*: Nil *PMH*: Back pain *DH*: Tramadol 50 mg QDS, Nurofen 200 mg TDS/PRN. *Information*: Last consultation for back pain 1 week ago with locum GP. You are a salaried GP.	*PC*: "I'm having trouble sleeping". *HPC*: Has difficulty getting to sleep and then wakes up several times in the night. Started approx 2 months ago. **Feels low in mood.** Rarely leaves the house now. No energy. **Some suicidal thoughts but no plans and his family would prevent him from doing this.** Poor concentration. No previous psychiatric problems. *ICE*: **Thinks low mood could be due to loneliness and also constant back pain. Poor support network.** *O/E*: Mental state examination – objectively and subjectively low mood. PHQ-9 score – 18/27.

Sleep disorders

- Up to 30% of the adult population have been affected by sleep problems at some time, especially the elderly.
- Problems include getting to sleep, staying asleep, waking too early, or disturbed sleep.
- Sleep problems can occur for various different reasons – medical reasons, emotional reasons, unhelpful surroundings or disturbed sleep routines.

Data gathering

Open question

- *"What problems have you been experiencing with your sleep?"*

Focused/closed questions

HPC: *"When did these problems first start?"*

"Do you have problems sleeping every day?"

"Are you aware of any particular triggers?"

"Do you have problems getting to sleep, staying asleep or waking too early?"

"When do you get to sleep at night?" "When do you wake up?" "Do you nap in the day?"

"Has your usual sleep routine or environment changed recently?"

"How is your general mood?"

PMH: Any history of depression or psychiatric problems?

Any medical conditions?

DH: Do you take any regular medications, e.g. stimulant medication?

"Have you tried any medication for your sleeping problem?"

SH: Who lives with you at home? Support network? Any relationship problems? Occupation? Stress at work? Smoking/alcohol/illicit drug history? Caffeine intake?

ICE: *"Do you have any idea what could be causing your sleeping problems?"*

"How is this sleep problem impacting on your daily life?"

Examination: • Nil specific.

Clinical management

Investigations

- Sleep diary and sleep studies.
- TFTs – if indicated from the history.

Management

- Avoid caffeine, alcohol and smoking in the evening.
- Ensure surroundings are amenable to sleep.

- Relaxation, e.g. bath before bedtime.
- Avoid napping during the day.
- Increase daytime exercise.
- Medications, e.g. anti-depressant if related to depression/anxiety (remember that sleeping tablets, for example, diazepam and zopiclone are addictive and ideally should not be given on a regular basis).

Role play

Information for doctor	Additional information for role player
Patient: Mrs EE *Age*: 76 years *SH*: Lives in a residential home. Retired. Non-smoker. No alcohol. *PMH*: Polymyalgia rheumatica *DH*: Prednisolone 5 mg daily. *Information*: Patient contacted the practice this morning requesting a home visit due to problems sleeping. You are a GP Registrar and have agreed to call her to find out further information.	*PC*: *"I'm having terrible trouble sleeping doctor".* *HPC*: Difficulty getting to sleep and also wakes up several times in the night. Problem started 6 months ago. Goes to bed at 10 pm and sleeps at 1 am. Feels very sleepy during the day. Mood fine. Drinks a lot of tea before bedtime. Goes to the toilet 2–3 times each night. *ICE*: Would like some sleeping tablets.

Deliberate self harm

- DSH describes acts such as self cutting or self poisoning, in which a patient deliberately causes harm or injury to themself, with or without suicidal intent.
- Self harm is most common in adolescence and early adulthood, and in those with psychiatric or personality disorders.
- Treatment includes psychological therapies and anti-depressant medications.

Data gathering

Open questions
- *"Can you tell me why you deliberately tried to harm yourself?"*
- *"Can you tell me more about what happened?"*

Focused/closed questions
HPC: *"Had you been planning this beforehand?"* (red flag)
"Did you write a suicide note beforehand?" (red flag)
"Did you plan it so that you wouldn't be found?" (red flag)
"How long have you been feeling this way for?"
"How did you feel whilst you were harming yourself?"

"How do you feel about it now? What is stopping you from harming yourself now?"

"Was it more of a cry for help or did you seriously want to end your life?"

"What will you do if you feel this way again?"

PMH: *"Have you ever tried to deliberately harm yourself before or have you ever tried to take your own life before?"* (red flag) Any past history of depression?

FH: Any family history of mental health problems or deliberate self harming?

DH: Do you currently take any regular medications? Anti-depressants? Anti-psychotics?

SH: Who lives with you at home? Occupation/School/College? Support network? Alcohol/smoking/illicit drug history?

ICE: *"What help would you like to prevent you from deliberately harming yourself again?"*

"How has your self harming affected your relationship with your family?"

Examination:
- Mental state examination (see *Appendix 3*).
- Physical examination relevant to specific self injury.

Clinical management

Investigations
- Risk assessment (consider red flags, e.g. psychiatric illness, suicidal intent, poor social support, drug abuse, risk of harm to self and others).

Explanation to patient
- There are many different reasons why people deliberately self harm, for example, to find relief from a terrible situation or as a way of coping with their emotions or feelings.
- There are a number of different methods that can be used to treat self harm and which concentrate on either treating the underlying causes or on treating the behaviour itself.

Management
(based on *NICE*, 2004, *CG16: Self-harm*)
- Urgently establish physical risk and mental state.
- Always offer physical treatment.
- Refer to A&E urgently if the patient is at significant risk of self injury.
- Support groups.
- Self-help guide www.patient.co.uk/health/Self-Harm-A-Self-Help-Guide.htm.
- Consider referral for psychological therapy.
- Consider anti-depressants if history of depression.
- Be vigilant when prescribing drugs to people who have previously self poisoned.
- Safety net – review again within the next week.

Role play

Information for doctor	Additional information for role player
Patient: Ms SW *Age*: 18 years *SH*: Lives with parents. College student. Smokes 10 cigs/day and also smokes cannabis. Drinks 30 units alcohol/ week. *PMH*: Depression, self harm; 2 previous hospital admissions. *DH*: Fluoxetine 20 mg daily *Information*: Was reviewed yesterday by the mental health crisis team after an episode of self harm. You are a GP Registrar.	*PC*: *"My mum wanted me to come to see you today because I self harmed yesterday"* *HPC*: *"I cut my wrists and arms".* **Superficial cuts. Felt fed up. Feels low. Parents were at home downstairs at the time.** No suicidal intent. Feels silly about it now. Didn't plan it beforehand. *FH*: No family history of mental illness. *ICE*: Poor eye contact. Subjective and objective low mood.

Post-traumatic stress disorder

- Condition where you have recurring distressing memories, flashbacks and nightmares after witnessing or suffering a traumatic event.
- Symptoms can develop soon after the trauma, or sometimes even months or years later.
- Other features include avoidance behaviour, hyperarousal or emotional numbing.

Data gathering

Open question
- *"Can you tell me more about what happened and how it is affecting you?"*

Focused/closed questions

HPC: *"Have you experienced a traumatic event?"*
"Have you been experiencing flashbacks or nightmares?"
"Have you been avoiding people or situations associated with the event?"
"Have you had problems sleeping or concentrating on things?"
"Have you been more irritable than usual?"
"Have you felt more detached from other people"
"Have you felt low in mood or unusually angry?"
"Have you had any thoughts of self harm or harming other people?" (red flags)
"Have you ever felt so low that you didn't want to carry on?" (red flag)

PMH: Any previous problems with depression or mental health issues?

DH: *"Are you on any regular medications?"*

SH: Occupation? Smoking/alcohol/illicit drug history

Examination: • Mental state examination (see *Appendix 3*).

Clinical management

Investigations

- Nil specific.

Explanation to patient

- It is normal to feel upset straight after a traumatic event, but for many people the distress gradually eases. If you have PTSD the distressing feelings and symptoms persist. In some cases the symptoms last a few months, and then ease or disappear. However, in some cases the symptoms persist long term.
- You may not need any treatment if your symptoms are mild. However, if your symptoms persist or are moderate or severe, treatment may be beneficial.

Management

(based on *NICE*, 2005, *CG26: Post-traumatic stress disorder*)

- If mild symptoms have been present for less than 4 weeks, manage with watchful waiting.
- All people with PTSD should be offered a course of trauma-focused CBT or eye movement desensitisation and reprocessing (EMDR).
- Drug treatments, e.g. paroxetine or mirtazapine, should be considered for the treatment of PTSD in adults who prefer not to have psychological therapy. It is not first line, however.
- Self help or support groups.
- Review regularly and if any red flags refer for specialist assessment and treatment.

Role play

Information for doctors	Additional information for role player
Patient: Mr AK *Age:* 42 years *SH:* Married, moved to UK 5 years ago from Iran. Works in internet café. Smokes 20 cigs/day. No alcohol intake or illicit drug use. Support network? *PMH:* Depression. *DH:* Mirtazapine 45 mg nocte *FH:* Nil *Information:* You are a GP Partner. You are reviewing this patient who first presented 2 weeks ago with flashbacks of being assaulted in Iran and sleeping difficulties.	*PC:* *"I have been suffering from bad nightmares doctor"* *HPC:* Was seriously assaulted 8 years ago in Iran. Has been having nightmares and sleeping problems for past year. First presentation. Too scared to go back to Iran. *ICE:* Doesn't feel able to work and is struggling financially. Would like sick note to claim benefits. *O/E:* Objectively and subjectively low mood. No visual or auditory hallucinations.

Cardiovascular

Angina pectoris

- Clinical syndrome characterised by discomfort usually in the chest, arm or jaw, precipitated by activities such as exercise which increase myocardial oxygen demand.
- Usually caused by coronary atherosclerosis, resulting in ischaemia of the heart vessels.
- Angina can be classified as stable or unstable:
  - Stable angina refers to a sensation of discomfort or pain in the chest, arm or jaw brought on by exertion, and relieved by rest or GTN.
  - Unstable angina is characterised by episodes of chest pain at rest, or increasingly rapidly with exertion, and which increase in frequency or severity. There is no ST elevation seen on an ECG.
- Risk factors for angina include hypertension, hypercholesterolaemia, smoking, physical inactivity and being overweight.

Data gathering

Open question
- *"Can you describe the chest pain that you have been experiencing?"*

Focused/closed questions
HPC: *"When did the pain first start?" "How frequently do you get the pain?"*
"How long does it last for?" (red flag if pain lasts >15 mins)
"Where do you feel the pain?"
"Does the pain spread anywhere else?"
"How would you describe the pain?"
"Do you get any pain at rest or on minimal exertion?" (red flag)
"How severe is the pain on a scale of 1 to 10?"
"Does anything make the pain better or worse?"
"Is the pain relieved by GTN spray?"
"Do you have any associated shortness of breath?"
"Do you wake up at night short of breath?" "How many pillows do you need to sleep with?"
"Have you noticed any nausea, clamminess or sensation that your heart is pounding?" (red flags)

PMH: Any previous heart problems? *"Any history of high blood pressure, high cholesterol or diabetes?"*
DH: Do you take any regular medications?
FH: Any family history of heart problems?
SH: Smoking/alcohol/illicit drug history? Occupation?
ICE: *"What do you think might be causing the chest pain?"*
Examination:
- BP, pulse.
- Cardiovascular system.

Clinical management

Investigations

- Blood test – FBC, U&Es, TFTs, LFTs, fasting glucose and cholesterol.
- ECG.
- Exercise test (or alternatively myocardial perfusion scintigraphy).
- Coronary angiogram – if high risk or unclear diagnosis.

Explanation to patient

- Angina describes the pain caused by narrowing of the heart arteries. There is a reduced blood supply to parts of the heart muscle.
- This blood supply may be enough to supply the heart when you are resting, but if you exert yourself the heart may not have enough blood and oxygen to function adequately.

Management

(based on *SIGN*, 2007, *96: Management of stable angina* and *NICE*, 2010, *CG95: Chest pain of recent onset*)

- If unstable angina, give 300 mg aspirin and immediate referral to hospital.
- Otherwise refer to the chest pain clinic for confirmation of the diagnosis and to assess the severity.
- Lifestyle modifications – stop smoking, treat high blood pressure, healthy diet, weight loss and exercise, reduce alcohol intake.
- Glyceryl trinitrate (GTN) used as required when the angina pain develops – relaxes the blood vessels reducing the load on the heart.
- Aspirin 75 mg daily and long term statin.
- Beta-blockers – first line drug, reduces the rate and force of the heart beat (if intolerant, alternatives include calcium channel blockers, long acting nitrates and nicorandil).
- Calcium channel blockers – second line.
- Refer to cardiology if symptoms not controlled despite maximum therapeutic doses of two drugs.
- ACE inhibitor – in patients with reduced LVF or with a past history of MI.
- Immunisations – pneumococcus and annual influenza.
- Inform DVLA (cannot hold an HGV licence).
- Safety net – seek medical attention immediately if red flag symptoms.

Role play

Information for doctor	Additional information for role player
Patient: Mr MK *Age*: 63 years *SH*: Lives with wife. Retired teacher. Never smoked. Alcohol 8 units/week. *PMH*: NIDDM, hypertension *DH*: Ramipril 2.5 mg OD, metformin 500 mg TDS, gliclazide 80 mg BD. *Information*: Saw nurse yesterday for BP check – 150/95. You are a locum GP.	*PC*: "*I have been getting some chest pain*." *HPC*: Chest pain only on moderate exertion. Pain in centre of chest with some radiation into the neck. **Pain lasts 1–2 mins each time. Rest relieves the pain. No palpitations, nausea or clamminess. Slight SOB with the pain.** *ICE*: Worried about his heart because is diabetic and has high blood pressure *O/E*: CVS exam – NAD.

Peripheral vascular disease

- Disease of the arteries whereby the arteries become narrowed, restricting blood flow to the muscles of the limbs. This can result in intermittent claudication.
- A common symptom is calf, buttock or thigh pain brought on by exercise and relieved by rest.
- Risk factors include smoking, obesity, inactivity, hypertension, diabetes and high cholesterol.

Data gathering

Open question
- "*Can you describe the pain in the calf that you've been experiencing?*"

Focused/closed questions
HPC: "*When did the problem first start?*"
"*Do you experience the pain at rest?*" (red flag)
"*How far can you walk before the onset of the pain?*"
"*Have you experienced any cramping of the legs?*"
"*Are both legs affected?*"
"*Have you noticed any colour changes in the foot?*" (red flag)
"*Have you noticed any swelling of your calves?*" (red flag)
"*Have you noticed any numbness in your leg?*" (red flag)
PMH: Any past history of heart disease? Any history of high blood pressure, high cholesterol or diabetes?
DH: Are you on any regular medications?
FH: Any family history of heart disease or diabetes?
SH: Smoking/alcohol/illicit drug history? Occupation? Stairs at home?

ICE: *"Does this problem stop you from doing things that you would normally be able to do?"*

Examination: • BP, pulse, weight.

• Cardiovascular system.

• Examination of leg – temperature, colour, peripheral pulses, inspection of skin.

Clinical management

Investigations
• Routine bloods – FBC, U&Es, fasting lipids and glucose.
• ECG.
• Ankle brachial pressure index.
• Doppler ultrasound scan.

Explanation to patient
• This is a narrowing of one or more arteries, and it mainly affects the arteries that supply blood to the legs. It is due to fatty plaques developing on the inside lining of the blood vessels.

Management
• Smoking cessation, exercise, weight loss, reduce alcohol intake.
• Foot care – regular self inspection and/or podiatry.
• Consider use of aspirin and statins.
• Treat any identifiable causes, e.g. hypertension, diabetes.
• Safety net – return if symptoms not improving or getting worse.
• Refer to vascular surgery urgently if rest pain, absent foot pulses, pallor or evidence of gangrene.

Role play

Information for doctor	Additional information for role player
Patient: Mr SA *Age*: 58 years *SH*: Lives alone. Widowed. Restaurant owner. Ex-smoker (20 pack years), no alcohol. *FH*: Nil *PMH*: MI 2004 *DH*: Aspirin 75 mg OD, simvastatin 40 mg nocte. *Information*: You are a salaried GP. Patient last seen 3 months ago for a medication review.	*PC*: Calf pain. *HPC*: 3 week history of bilateral calf pain brought on by exertion and relieved by rest. **No rest pain. Pain brought on after 200 m walking. No SOB or chest pain. No swelling of the calves.** No leg swelling. No colour changes in the foot or lower leg. *ICE*: Would like to know what is causing the pain. Unable to go out much due to this pain. *O/E*: BP 150/90. HR 75, regular. CVS exam – NAD. Calves soft, non-tender. No calf swelling bilaterally. Legs pale and cool bilaterally. Diminished foot pulses.

Palpitations

- Awareness of your own heartbeat.
- Can be caused by cardiac problems, for example, atrial fibrillation, or from anxiety.
- Requires urgent referral if suspected or proven ventricular tachycardia.

Data gathering

Open questions
- *"Can you describe in more detail the palpitations you have been experiencing?"*
- *"What do you mean by palpitations?"*

Focused/closed questions

HPC: *"When did you first start being aware of your own heartbeat?"*
"How frequently is this occurring?" "How long does it last for?"
"Do you feel your heart beating regularly or irregularly?"
"Could you tap out the rhythm of your heartbeat on the table?"
"Have you noticed any associated shortness of breath or chest pain?"
(red flags)
"Do you have any episodes of dizziness, clamminess or collapse?"
(red flags)
"How much caffeine do you drink on a daily basis?"
"Have you been feeling more anxious than usual?"
"Do you have a fever?"
"Have you been feeling more tired than usual?"
"Any changes to your weight?"

PMH: Any history of anxiety or previous heart problems?

DH: Do you take any regular medications? (e.g. bronchodilators, amlodipine, levothyroxine or withdrawal from benzodiazepines can cause palpitations) Have you been taking any cold decongestants?

FH: Any family history of heart problems, thyroid problems, anxiety or unexplained death?

SH: Alcohol/smoking/illicit drug history? (cocaine and amphetamines can cause palpitations). Occupation? Stress?

ICE: *"What particularly concerned you about these palpitations?"*

Examination:
- BP, pulse.
- Check for anaemia.
- CVS examination.
- Thyroid examination – if any other symptoms.

Clinical management

Investigations

- 12-lead ECG.
- 24 hour ECG.
- Blood test – FBC, U&Es and TFTs, glucose and cholesterol.

Explanation to patient

- Unpleasant awareness of your heartbeat, often described as thumping in your chest.

Management

- Arrange emergency admission for anyone with palpitations with VT or SVT or if additional symptoms of chest pain, SOB or syncope.
- If sinus tachycardia +/– ectopic beats with no adverse features, e.g. structural heart disease, reassure and advise on lifestyle, caffeine and alcohol. If any adverse features, refer to secondary care.
- If AF (chronic or paroxysmal) – refer to NICE guidelines (2006, *CG36: Atrial fibrillation*).
- If related to anxiety, advise self help measures.
- Notify DVLA if associated syncope or cardiac cause.
- Safety net – if palpitations not resolving, return to the GP.

Role play

Information for doctors	Additional information for role player
Patient: Mr JB *Age*: 24 years *SH*: University student, lives in shared flat *PMH*: Depression *FH*: Mother and sister have anxiety. *DH*: Fluoxetine 20 mg OD *Information*: Last saw GP 1 week ago for medication review. You are a locum GP.	*PC*: Palpitations. *HPC*: Started experiencing palpitations intermittently since last week. Gets palpitations 2–3× daily. **Fast heart beat but seems regular. Slight SOB also.** No chest pain. Has been under stress recently with university exams. No dizziness or clamminess. Currently drinks 5–6 cups of coffee each day. Smokes 10 cigs/day. *ICE*: **Worried about his heart.** *O/E*: BP 110/60, CV and respiratory exam – NAD. HR 82, regular.

Respiratory

Asthma

- Common condition affecting the airways of the lungs, resulting in typical symptoms of wheeze, cough, chest tightness and shortness of breath.
- Diagnosis is based on recognition of characteristic pattern of signs and symptoms and measurement of airflow obstruction.
- Treatment is usually with inhalers – typically a bronchodilator and/or corticosteroids.

Data gathering

Open question
- *"Can you tell me more about the problems with your breathing?"*

Focused/closed questions

HPC: *"How long have you been experiencing these symptoms for?"*
"Does anything make your breathing better or worse, e.g. cold weather, certain medications or exercise?"
"Do you have a cough, wheeze, shortness of breath, or chest tightness?"
"Is the cough or wheeze worse at any particular time of the day?"
"How regularly do you use your inhalers?" (red flag if uncontrolled symptoms)
"Do you know how to use your inhalers correctly?"
"Have you required any oral steroids in the past year due to breathing problems?" *"If so, how many?"*

PMH: Any past history of breathing problems? Any previous asthma attacks or hospital admissions due to asthma? Any ITU admissions?

FH: Any family history of asthma, eczema or hayfever?

DH: What medications are you currently taking, e.g. inhalers? *"How often do you use your inhalers?"* *"Do you use a spacer device?"*

SH: Smoking history? Occupation? Any damp or dust in your home? Any pets?

ICE: *"What were you hoping we could do to help with this breathing problem?"*
"How does this problem affect you at home/school/work?"

Examination:
- Respiratory examination (red flag if respiratory distress or silent chest).

- Peak flow.
- Inhaler/spacer technique.

Clinical management

Investigations
- Spirometry (diagnosis of asthma is likely if FEV_1/FVC <70%).
- Reversibility testing (expect 15% improvement in PEFR after trial of bronchodilator).
- PEFR diary.
- CXR – if unclear diagnosis.

Explanation to patient
- A condition affecting the airways of the lungs. The muscles around the walls of the airway tighten so that the airway becomes narrower. The lining of the airways also becomes inflamed and this makes it difficult to breathe, resulting in the symptoms of asthma.

Management
(based on *BTS/ SIGN*, 2014, *British guideline on the management of asthma*)
- Lifestyle measures – weight loss, smoking cessation, allergen avoidance, breathing exercises.
- Education on self management including personalised asthma action plan.
- If high probability of asthma (FEV_1/FVC <70%), arrange trial of asthma treatment.
- Stepwise management in adults
  1. Inhaled short-acting beta agonist e.g. salbutamol, PRN.
  2. Add inhaled corticosteroid 200–800 mcg/day.
  3. Add inhaled long-acting beta agonist (LABA), e.g. salmeterol. If good response to LABA but control still inadequate, increase the inhaled steroid. If no response to LABA stop this and increase the inhaled steroid.
  4. Add leucotriene receptor antagonist or SR theophylline.
  5. Increase inhaled corticosteroid up to 2000 mcg daily if persistent poor control.
  6. Use daily steroid tablet in lowest dose if frequent use of oral steroids.
- Admit patients immediately with any features of life threatening asthma or severe asthma not responding to initial treatment.
- Safety net – arrange follow-up to review progress, based on severity of symptoms.
- Step down, when control is good, should be done at 3-monthly intervals.

Role play

Information for doctor	Additional information for role player
Patient: Mr JA *Age*: 19 years *SH*: College student, lives with parents. Non-smoker. *FH*: Mother and sister have asthma and eczema *PMH*: Asthma. No previous hospital admissions *DH*: Salbutamol 1–2 puffs PRN, beclomethasone 2 puffs BD *Information*: Asthma review with nurse 1 week ago – peak flow 250 l/min. You are a salaried GP.	*PC*: Worsening symptoms of asthma, requiring salbutamol several times a day. *HPC*: **Waking at night with cough and chest tightness.** Unable to participate in sports due to breathing problems. Wheeze also. Using salbutamol 6× daily and beclomethasone twice daily. *ICE*: Concerned about not being able to participate in sports as was previously very active and enjoys sports. *O/E*: Chest – bilateral equal air entry. Generalised wheeze throughout both lung fields. Poor inhaler technique.

Chronic obstructive pulmonary disease

- COPD (otherwise referred to as emphysema or bronchitis) is characterised by airflow obstruction which is usually progressive and not fully reversible.
- With emphysema the air sacs of the lungs are gradually destroyed, resulting in difficulty absorbing enough oxygen.
- With chronic bronchitis the airways become narrower, and there is increased mucus production and inflammation.
- A diagnosis of COPD should be considered in those aged over 35 years who are smokers or ex-smokers and who have exertional breathlessness, chronic cough, wheeze or regular sputum production.

Data gathering

Open question
- *"Can you tell me more about your breathing problems?"*

Focused/closed questions
HPC: *"Do you have a cough, sputum production, wheeze or any shortness of breath?"*
"How long have you had a cough for?"
"Do you ever get short of breath at rest?" (red flag)
"Have you been coughing up any phlegm?" *"If so, what colour is it?"*
"Do you get recurrent 'winter bronchitis'?"

"Have you noticed any weight loss or blood when you cough?" (red flag)
"Do you have any chest pain?" (red flag)
"Do you have any ankle swelling or do you wake at night short of breath?" (red flag)
"How frequently do you suffer with chest infections?"

PMH: Any previous chest problems? Any previous hospital admissions due to chest problems?

DH: Regular medications? Inhalers?

FH: Any FH of chest problems?

SH: Smoking history? Occupation? Who lives with you at home? How do you manage at home?

ICE: *"How is your breathing affecting your daily activities?"*

Examination:
- BMI.
- Oxygen saturations.
- Respiratory examination.
- Inhaler technique.

Clinical management

Investigation
- CXR – to exclude other causes.
- Spirometry (COPD is defined as FEV/FVC <70% PLUS FEV <80% or FEV >80% in the presence of SOB or cough).
- Determine severity of airflow obstruction (mild COPD = FEV_1 >80%, moderate COPD = FEV_1 50–80%, severe COPD = FEV_1 30–49%, very severe COPD = FEV_1 <30%).
- FBC (to identify anaemia or polycythaemia).

Explanation to patient
- COPD describes obstruction of the airways that is not reversible. It is often caused by smoking. Inhalers are used to ease the symptoms. Stopping smoking is the single most effective treatment.

Management
(based on *NICE, 2010, CG101: Chronic obstructive pulmonary disease (update)*)
- Lifestyle measures – smoking cessation, weight loss, exercise.
- Stepwise management:
  1. Short-acting beta agonist, e.g. salbutamol. Ipratropium is no longer recommended as it may increase CVD risk.
  2. Add long-acting beta agonist (LABA), e.g. salmeterol, or long-acting muscarinic agonist (LAMA), e.g. tiotropium. Handihaler is recommended over mist inhaler. Add inhaled corticosteroid (ICS) in combination with these if FEV_1<50%, although there is an increased risk of pneumonia with ICS so patients should be made aware of this.
  3. Trial of theophylline.

- Mucolytic drugs – if chronic productive cough.
- Consider long term oxygen therapy if FEV_1 <50% or O_2 sats <92% in air.
- Refer to specialist if diagnostic uncertainty, suspected severe COPD, rapid decline in FEV_1, frequent infections or for consideration of long term oxygen therapy.
- Review people with mild–moderate COPD at least once a year and those with severe COPD at least twice yearly.
- Offer pneumococcal and annual influenza vaccinations.
- Treatment of exacerbations:
  - Increase frequency of bronchodilators and give oral antibiotic if purulent sputum or clinical signs of infection.
  - Offer prednisolone 40 mg daily for 5 days.
  - Safety net – arrange to review and inform patient what to do if symptoms worsen.

Role play

Information for doctor	Additional information for role player
Patient: Mr RM *Age*: 52 years *SH*: Lives with wife. Unemployed. Ex-smoker (20 pack years). *FH*: Nil *PMH*: COPD *DH*: Ipratropium 500 mcg QDS and tiotropium 5 mcg OD. *Information*: Had annual COPD review with nurse yesterday: FEV_1 – 48% FEV_1/FVC – 0.5. You are a GP Partner.	*PC*: *"I feel more breathless even though I'm taking my inhalers regularly".* *HPC*: SOB even with minimal exertion (walking a few yards). Cough with clear sputum production. No recent weight loss. No chest pain. **No haemoptysis. No ankle swelling.** Last chest infection 6 months ago. *PMH*: No previous hospital admissions with COPD. *ICE*: Worried about worsening COPD. *O/E*: BMI 26. Bilateral equal air entry. Widespread wheeze bilaterally.

Gastrointestinal and renal

Dyspepsia

- Symptoms related to problems with digestion.
- Common symptoms include epigastric pain, bloating, nausea or vomiting.
- Causes include 'functional' dyspepsia, duodenal and gastric ulcers, oesophagitis, gastritis, gastro-oesophageal reflux and *Helicobacter pylori* infection.
- Management includes avoidance of triggers, antacids or acid suppressing medication.

Data gathering

Open question

- *"Can you tell me more about these symptoms?"*

Focused/closed questions

HPC: *"Any abdominal pain/nausea/bloating/vomiting?"*
"When did the problem first start?"
"How often do you experience these symptoms?"
"Do you know what triggers the symptoms?"
"Is the problem worse at night or after eating?"
"Any abdominal pain/ nausea/ bloating/ vomiting?"
"Any bleeding from the back passage, vomiting blood or weight loss?" (red flags)
"Any difficulties swallowing?"

PMH: Any previous stomach problems? Any previous *H. pylori* infection?

FH Any family history of stomach problems?

DH: Do you take any regular medications? NSAIDs/calcium antagonists/bisphosphonates?

SH: Occupation? Stress? Smoking/alcohol/illicit drug history?

ICE: *"Do you have any thoughts as to what is causing these symptoms?"*

Examination: • Abdominal examination.

Clinical management

Investigations

- Bloods – FBC, ferritin, LFTs, coeliac screen.

- *H. pylori* test (either stool antigen, carbon-13 urea breath test or lab-based serology). Serology is not recommended for the elderly, children or post-treatment.
- Referral for upper GI endoscopy in resistant cases. Avoid PPIs or H_2 receptor blockers for at least 2 weeks beforehand.
- NICE (2014, *CG184: Dyspepsia and GORD*). Refer for urgent endoscopy if dyspepsia and one or more alarm symptoms at any age.

Explanation to patient

- Dyspepsia (or indigestion) describes the symptoms that occur when there is a problem with the digestion in the upper gut. Abdominal pain and bloating are common symptoms, and it may be caused by certain medications, for example anti-inflammatory drugs, or by eating certain types of food, for example spicy foods.

Management

- Conservative management – stop smoking, weight loss, avoidance of spicy foods and alcohol, caffeine reduction.
- Antacids (e.g. Gaviscon) – neutralises stomach acid.
- Stop or change any medications thought to be triggering symptoms, e.g. NSAIDs, steroids, nitrates or bisphosphonates.
- Acid suppressing medication, e.g. proton pump inhibitors (omeprazole/ lansoprazole) or H_2 receptor blockers.
- Offer full dose PPI for 4 weeks or the *H. pylori* 'test and treat' can be done for people with dyspepsia / reflux and no red flag symptoms (*NICE*, 2014, *CG184: Dyspepsia and GORD*).
- Safety net – review in 6 weeks if symptoms not improving, or sooner if there is a deterioration in symptoms.

Role play

Information for doctor		Additional information for role player
Patient:	Mr TP	*PC*: "*I've been getting terrible indigestion, and Gaviscon isn't helping*"
Age:	54 years	*HPC*: Pain in upper abdomen sometimes spreading into the chest. Started 3 weeks ago and occurs 2–3 times daily. **Worse at night and after eating. Some bloating. No obvious food triggers. No vomiting, haematemesis, melaena or weight loss. No dysphagia.**
SH:	Lives with wife. Taxi driver. Smokes 20 cigs/day. Drinks 50 units alcohol/ week.	
PMH:	Hypercholesterolaemia	
DH:	Simvastatin 40 mg nocte	*ICE*: Would like some stronger medication as his friend has a similar problem and was given something from his doctor.
Information:	You are a GP Registrar.	*O/E*: Soft abdomen. Mild epigastric tenderness. No palpable masses or organomegaly.

Rectal bleeding

- Refers to gastrointestinal tract bleeding.
- Causes include haemorrhoids, anal fissures, diverticular disease, inflammatory bowel disease or bowel cancer.
- A colonoscopy may be recommended to confirm the diagnosis.

Data gathering

Open question

- *"Can you tell me more about the bleeding from your back passage?"*

Focused/closed questions

HPC: *"When did the bleeding from your back passage start?"*
"Is the blood mixed in with the stool or on the toilet paper?"
"Is the blood bright red or is it darker?"
"Have you noticed any weight loss?" (red flag)
"Any change in bowel habit?" (red flag)
"Any itchiness or soreness around the back passage?"
"Have you passed any mucus in the stools?"
"Are you aware of any abdominal pain?"
"Do you have any pain around your back passage?"
"Have you noticed any dizziness or fatigue?"
"Have you had an associated fever?"
"Are you constipated?"

PMH: *"Have you had any previous bowel problems or episodes of rectal bleeding?"*

DH: Do you take any regular medications, e.g. warfarin or NSAIDs?

FH: Any family history of bowel problems or bowel cancer?

SH: Smoking/alcohol/illicit drug history?

ICE: *"Do you have any concerns about what might be causing the rectal bleeding?"*

Examination:
- BP, pulse and temperature.
- Gastrointestinal examination including digital rectal examination.

Clinical management

Investigations

- Blood test – FBC, ferritin, U&Es, CRP, LFTs, clotting studies.
- Faecal occult blood test.
- Colonoscopy or sigmoidoscopy.

Explanation to patient
- Blood appearing from the back passage.
- Most episodes of rectal bleeding are mild and stop on their own.
- Sometimes a small telescope with a camera attached is inserted into the back passage to investigate the cause of the bleeding.

Management
- Determined by the diagnosis.
- If any signs of shock or melaena, refer to A&E immediately.
- Refer for suspected cancer under the two week wait if:
  - Aged under 50 with rectal bleeding and any of the following unexplained symptoms – abdominal pain, change in bowel habit, weight loss or iron deficiency anaemia.
  - Aged 40 or over with unexplained weight loss and abdominal pain.
  - Aged 60 or over with iron deficiency anaemia or changes in their bowel habit or a positive faecal occult blood test.
- Safety net – if symptoms not improving return to GP.

Role play

Information for doctor	Additional information for role player
Patient: Mr OM *Age*: 34 years *SH*: Lives alone. University lecturer. Non smoker. *FH*: Father and paternal grandmother – diabetes. *PMH*: Nil *DH*: Nil *Information*: No previous consultations. You are a GP Partner.	*PC*: "*I've been passing blood when I go to the toilet*". *HPC*: Six week history of diarrhoea with fresh blood in the stools. **Approx 5 kg weight loss. Also lower abdominal pain when opening bowels. Bowels opening approx 3 times daily. Blood mixed in stools.** *ICE*: Very worried about cancer. Has been putting off coming to the doctor. *O/E*: BP 110/70. HR 70. Pallor; abdomen tender in LIF. No palpable masses. Rectal examination – fresh blood, no masses.

Anaemia

- Fewer red blood cells than normal or less haemoglobin than normal in each red blood cell.
- This results in a reduced amount of oxygen being carried around in the blood stream.
- Symptoms include tiredness, lethargy, dizziness, SOB, and headaches.
- Causes include iron deficiency anaemia, haemoglobinopathies, anaemia of chronic disease and B_{12} deficiency.

Data gathering

Open question

- *"Can you tell me what symptoms you have been experiencing?"*

Focused/closed questions

HPC: *"Have you been experiencing any tiredness, dizziness, breathlessness or headaches?"*

"Have you noticed any change in your appetite?"

"Have you experienced any chest pain?" (red flag)

"Have you felt a sensation of your heart pounding?"

"Has anyone commented that you look paler than usual?"

"Are your periods heavier than usual?"

"Have you noticed any blood in the stools or in the urine?" (red flags)

"Have you noticed any change to your bowel habit or weight loss?" (red flags)

"Have you coughed up any blood?" (red flag)

"Do you have a well balanced diet with a variety of meats and vegetables?"

"Have you noticed any bruising or bone pains?" (red flags)

"Have you had any vomiting or abdominal pain?"

PMH: Any other medical conditions?

DH: Do you take any regular medications, e.g. warfarin, NSAIDs?

SH: Smoking/alcohol/illicit drug history? Occupation? Who lives with you at home?

FH: Any family history of anaemia or any blood disorders?

ICE: "What do you think is causing your anaemia?"

Examination:
- Check for pale conjunctiva, pallor, gum hypertrophy, and koilonychia.
- BP and pulse.
- Cardiovascular system – check for systolic ejection murmur.
- Abdominal examination – if suspected GI cause.

Clinical management

Investigations

- Blood tests – FBC, ferritin, B$_{12}$, folate, blood film, haemoglobin electrophoresis, LFTs, TFTs and coeliac screen.
- Faecal occult blood – to determine if any GI blood loss.
- Endoscopy or colonoscopy – if required to determine site of blood loss.

Explanation to patient

- Red blood cells carry oxygen around the body in a substance called haemoglobin. Haemoglobin gives your blood its red colour. Iron is an important part of haemoglobin.
- If you don't have enough red blood cells, or enough of the oxygen-carrying substance haemoglobin, you have anaemia.

- Anaemia can result from an increased loss or rate of destruction of red blood cells or decreased production of red blood cells.

Management

(based on *NHS CKS*, 2008, *Anaemia – iron deficiency – management*)

- Address underlying cause, e.g. menorrhagia, stopping NSAIDs.
- Increase dietary intake of iron (red meat, green vegetables, pulses), vitamin B_{12} (meat, milk, cheese, eggs) and folate (liver, yeast extract, green leafy vegetables).
- Vitamin supplements.
- Ferrous sulphate 200 mg two to three times daily – if iron deficiency anaemia.
- Vitamin B_{12} injections – if vitamin B_{12} deficient (refer urgently to specialist if any neurological involvement or if pregnant).
- Refer to specialist if unexplained iron deficiency anaemia.
- Refer for blood transfusion if Hb <7 and symptomatic.
- Safety net – return to GP if symptoms no better after 2–4 weeks.

Role play

Information for doctor	Additional information for role player
Patient: Ms BN *Age*: 25 years *SH*: Lives with boyfriend and 18 month old baby. Hairdresser. Alcohol 15 units/week. Non smoker. *PMH*: Nil *DH*: Nil *Information*: Last consultation with GP for IUCD insertion 6 months ago. You are a salaried GP.	*PC*: "*My boyfriend thinks I look paler than usual, so I wanted to check if I'm anaemic*". *HPC*: Has felt more tired than usual for past month. **Periods have been heavier**. **Negative pregnancy test**. No SOB. No dizziness or headache. No weight loss. No change in bowel habit or blood in stools/urine. Had anaemia in pregnancy previously. **Vegetarian – eats lots of green vegetables.** *ICE*: Having difficulty going to work due to tiredness and low energy levels. *O/E*: Pallor. BP 100/60. HR 60, regular. Abdominal examination – NAD. Pelvic/speculum exam – IUCD threads visible.

Coeliac disease

- Coeliac disease is believed to be present in up to 1 in 100 of the population, although only about 10–15% of people with the condition are clinically diagnosed.
- It is important to identify people with undiagnosed disease because it can be treated effectively with a gluten-free diet.
- Non-coeliac gluten sensitivity is now a recognised condition also.

Data gathering

Open question

- "*Can you tell me a bit more about your symptoms?*"

Focused/closed question

HPC: *"Have you had any diarrhoea or vomiting?"*
"Have you had any abdominal pain?"
"Have you been bloated?"
"Have you noticed any change to your weight?"
"Have you been feeling more tired than usual?"

PMH: *"Do you have any medical conditions, for example, diabetes or a thyroid disorder?"*

DH: *"Do you take any regular medications?"*

FH: *"Is there a family history of any bowel problems, for example coeliac disease?"*

SH: *"Who lives with you at home?"* Smoking/alcohol/drugs

ICE: *"What concerns do you have with regards to your symptoms?"*

Examination:
- BMI.
- Abdominal examination – pallor, abdominal distension, abdominal tenderness.

Clinical management

(based on *NICE*, 2009, *CG86: Coeliac disease*)

Investigations
- Stool MC&S.
- Blood test – FBC, U&Es, LFTs, ESR, calcium, IgA tissue transglutaminase*.
- Endoscopy and intestinal biopsy if positive serology. Consider also if serology negative but coeliac remains clinically suspected.

*First line serological test (can use IgA endomysial antibodies if this is equivocal).

Explanation to patient
- Coeliac disease is a condition mainly affecting part of the bowel. It is caused by a reaction of the bowel to gluten, which is found mainly in foods made from wheat, barley and rye.
- Inflammation occurs in the lining of the small intestine resulting in food not being properly absorbed. Symptoms such as bloating, abdominal pain, diarrhoea and weight loss result.
- If the blood test to check for coeliac disease is positive, a sample of the small bowel will need to be taken to confirm the diagnosis.
- If coeliac disease is confirmed you will be required to follow a gluten-free diet.

Management
- Lifelong gluten-free diet.
- Dietitian referral.
- Vitamin supplements at least for first 6 months – iron and calcium.
- In patients with persistent abdominal symptoms and negative tests consider trialling a 4-week gluten-free diet.

- Annual blood tests – FBC, ferritin, B_{12}, folate, calcium, vitamin D, glucose, TSH, Igs, tTGA. Consider LFTs also.
- Offer haemophilus, flu, men C and pneumococcal vaccinations.
- Initial 3–6 monthly follow up.

Role play

Information for doctor	Additional information for role player
Patient: Miss RJ *Age*: 19 years *PMH*: IBS *DH*: Loperamide 4 mg BD/PRN, buscopan 10 mg TDS. *FH*: Mother has IBS. Grandmother has NIDDM. *Information*: You are a GP Partner. You have seen this patient several times recently with diarrhoea symptoms. She has come today to discuss her blood test results: Hb 12.1; WCC 4.8; ESR 12; IgA tTGA positive. LFTs NAD.	*PC*: "*I have come today for my blood test results*" *HPC*: 6 month history of worsening diarrhoea approx 3× daily. No blood or mucus in stools. Also abdo bloating and tiredness. Some mild generalised abdo pain. No vomiting. 5 kg weight loss over past 6 months. *ICE*: Worried that her IBS is not well controlled. *O/E*: BMI 19. Abdo examination – abdominal distension and mild generalised tenderness. Pallor.

Irritable bowel syndrome

- IBS is a common disorder affecting the digestive system due to a problem with the function of the gut.
- Symptoms include abdominal pain, diarrhoea, constipation and bloating.
- Approximately 10–20% of people will be affected by IBS at any one time in the UK (*NICE*, 2008, *CG61: Irritable bowel syndrome*).
- Treatment includes dietary advice, antispasmodic medication, constipation medication or psychological therapy.

Data gathering

Open question
- "*Can you tell me about the bowel symptoms you have been experiencing?*"

Focused/closed questions
HPC: "*Do you have any abdominal pain or bloating?*"
"*Where exactly is the abdominal pain?*"
"*How long have you had these symptoms for?*"
"*Is the abdominal pain relieved by opening your bowels?*"
"*Have you noticed a change in your bowel habit, weight loss or bleeding from your back passage?*" (red flags)
"*Are you troubled by these symptoms at night?*" (red flag)
"*Have you passed any mucus in your stools?*"

"Have you been straining to pass stools or alternatively do you ever have an urgency to open your bowels?"

"Are your symptoms worse after eating?"

PMH: Any previous history of bowel problems? Any previous operations on your bowel?

FH: Any FH of bowel problems?

DH: Are you taking any regular medications?

SH: Smoking/alcohol history? Occupation?

ICE: *"Do you have any particular concerns about your bowel problems?"*

Examination:
- BMI.
- Abdominal examination.
- Rectal examination (to check for masses and any blood in stools).
- Consider pelvic examination if any suspicion of ovarian cancer.

Clinical management

Investigations
- Blood test (FBC, ESR, CRP, endomysial antibodies (EMA) or tissue transglutaminase (TTG) for coeliac disease).
- Faecal calprotectin – useful diagnostic tool to exclude IBD in patients with suspected IBS.
- Colonoscopy – if need to rule out bowel cancer, but is not a routine investigation if suspecting IBS.

Explanation to patient
- IBS is a condition affecting the function of the gut. It is thought that there may be over-activity of part of the bowel.

Management
(based on *NICE*, 2008, *CG61: Irritable bowel syndrome*)
- Reassurance – does not lead to bowel cancer.
- Symptom diary.
- Regular meals and at least 8 glasses of water/fluid daily.
- Restrict tea/coffee/fizzy drinks/alcohol.
- Limit fresh fruit and high fibre food.
- Low FODMAP diet – when general lifestyle and dietary measures have not relieved symptoms.
- Consider trial of daily supplementation with linseeds or trial of probiotics.
- Regular exercise.
- Medications – e.g. buscopan, lactulose, loperamide, tricyclic anti-depressants. Linaclotide is a new treatment available but is pricey.
- Safety net – review again if symptoms not improving after 4–6 weeks or if any red flag symptoms.
- For those whose symptoms don't improve after 12 months, consider referring for psychological therapies.

Role play

Information for doctor	Additional information for role player
Patient: Mrs JJ *Age*: 37 years *SH*: Married, 2 children, housewife *PMH*: Asthma *DH*: Salbutamol 1–2 puffs PRN *Information*: Last consultation 6 months ago due to diarrhoea. No infective cause found. You are a locum GP.	*PC*: *"I've been having problems with my bowels".* *HPC*: Intermittent diarrhoea/constipation for the past month. Some bloating. **No rectal bleeding.** Intermittent lower abdominal pain. No weight loss or mucus in stools. Hasn't tried any medications so far. Drinks 4 cups coffee per day and has a lot of fibre in her diet. *FH*: Nil. *ICE*: Would like referral to the specialist. *O/E*: BMI 30. Abdo exam and rectal exam – NAD.

Gallstones

- Small stones, usually made of cholesterol, which form in the gallbladder.
- Approximately 1 in 3 women and 1 in 6 men will have gallstones at some stage in their lifetime.
- The figure below shows a simple diagram of the gallbladder that can be used to help explain gallstones to your patient.

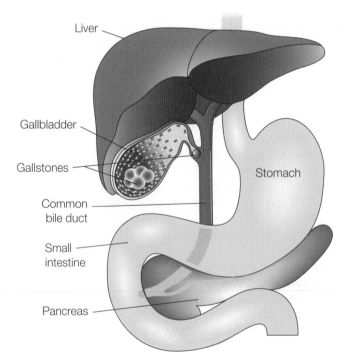

Data gathering

Open question
- *"Can you tell me more about the abdominal pain you've been experiencing?"*

Focused/closed questions

HPC: *"Where exactly is the pain?" "Does it spread anywhere else?" "When did it first start?"*
"What type of pain is it?" "Is the pain intermittent or constant?"
"Does anything make the pain better or worse?" "Do any particular foods make the pain worse?"
"Have you had any vomiting or nausea?"
"Have you had any fever?" (red flag)
"Have you had any episodes of severe abdominal pain?" "If so, how long did it last for?"
"Any weight loss or vomiting of blood?" (red flags)
"Have you ever noticed a yellow discoloration of your skin?" (red flag)

PMH: Any significant medical history?

DH: Are you taking any regular medications? Have you tried any medications to help with the abdominal pain?

FH: Any family history of gallstones or gastrointestinal problems?

SH: Smoking/alcohol/illicit drug history? Occupation?

ICE: *"Do you have any idea what might be causing this abdominal pain?"*
"How does this pain affect you from day to day?"

Examination:
- Temperature, pulse and BP.
- Abdominal examination (including Murphy's sign).

Clinical management

Investigations
- Blood tests – FBC, U&Es, LFTs, CRP, ESR.
- Abdominal ultrasound scan.

Explanation to patient
- Gallstones are formed when some of the chemicals stored in the gallbladder harden to form a mass. It can form one big stone or lots of tiny stones.
- In most cases, gallstones do not cause any symptoms.
- In a small number of cases, gallstones can lead to symptoms due to the stones either becoming trapped in a duct, causing inflammation of the gallbladder, or by moving out into other parts of the body resulting in pain, jaundice (yellow discoloration of the skin) or inflammation of the pancreas.

Management
- Leave alone if causes few or no symptoms.

- Ursodeoxycholic acid – can sometimes dissolve small stones although not commonly used.
- Safety net – review again within 2–3 weeks if symptoms not improving, or sooner if symptoms worsening or the patient develops fever.
- Surgery – cholecystectomy.

Role play

Information for doctor	Additional information for role player
Patient: Mrs CP *Age*: 44 years *SH*: Married, smokes 15 cigs/day, 20 units alcohol/wk. Accountant. *PMH*: Dyspepsia *DH*: Omeprazole 40 mg daily *Information*: Was seen last night by OOH service due to RUQ pain. Was given pain relief and advised to see GP today.	*PC*: Abdominal pain. *HPC*: Intermittent sharp RUQ pain for past few days, which has increased in severity since last night. One episode of vomiting. No fever. Co-codamol helps with the pain. **Pain worse after eating fatty foods. No jaundice.** *ICE*: **Worried about what is causing the pain. Would like a scan done.** *O/E*: BMI 32. Abdomen soft, RUQ tenderness. No guarding. No organomegaly or palpable masses. Murphy's sign positive.

Chronic kidney disease

- CKD is a common problem which is often sub-optimally managed and about which patients are inadequately informed (*BJGP*, 2012; 62: 184).
- Those at higher risk of developing CKD should be offered routine testing, including patients with diabetes, hypertension, cardiovascular disease, structural renal tract disease or those prescribed nephrotoxic drugs (*NICE*, 2014, *CKD guideline*).
- The NICE 2014 guideline introduces fundamental changes to practice, including new definitions and classifications of CKD and the use of the cystatin C test.
- CKD is now defined using G (eGFR) and A (albumin creatinine ratio) criteria.

GFR category	GFR
G1	>90 (normal)
G2	60–89
G3a	45–59
G3b	30–44
G4	15–29
G5	<15 (kidney failure)

Urine ACR categories:	
ACR category	*ACR (mg/mmol)*
A1	<3
A2	3–30
A3	>30

Data gathering

Open questions
- *"What problems have you been experiencing with your kidneys?"*
- *"Can you tell me more about your symptoms?"*

Focused/closed questions

HPC: *"Have you felt more tired than usual?"*
"Have you noticed any blood in your urine?"
"How many times do you get up at night to pass urine?"
"Have you been passing more urine than usual?"
"Have you noticed any swelling of your feet or ankles?"
"Have you had any shortness of breath, nausea or vomiting?"
"Have you noticed that your skin is more itchy than usual?"
"Have you noticed any weight loss?" (red flag)
"Have you noticed any change in your appetite?"

PMH: Do you have high blood pressure or diabetes? Have you had any previous problems with your kidneys or heart?

DH: Do you take any regular medications?
NSAIDs/ACE inhibitors/diuretics?

FH: Any family history of kidney problems?

SH: Smoking/alcohol/illicit drug history? Occupation? Who lives with you at home?

ICE: *"What do you think is causing your symptoms?"*

Examination:
- BP.
- Weight.
- Check for anaemia and uraemia.
- Abdominal examination including palpation of kidneys.

Clinical management

Investigations
- Blood test – FBC, U&Es, LFTs, eGFR, calcium, phosphate, fasting glucose and lipids, HIV/Hep B serology, autoantibodies.
- Check urine for proteinuria (ACR), blood and MC&S.
- Renal ultrasound scan.
- Renal biopsy or CT/MRI in secondary care.

Explanation to patient
- The kidneys are two bean-shaped organs which filter out waste products from the blood before converting them into urine. They also help to maintain blood pressure and produce a substance which stimulates red blood cell production.
- Over time, the kidneys become less efficient and this is made worse by diabetes and high blood pressure.

Management

(based on *NICE, 2014, CKD guideline*)

- General lifestyle advice – achieve a healthy weight, exercise, stop smoking, low salt diet, avoid nephrotoxic drugs.
- Aim to keep BP well controlled (consider using ACE inhibitors or angiotensin receptor blockers). Ideally BP should be below 140/90 (or <130/80 if diabetic).
- Reduce CV disease risk (consider statins and antiplatelets).
- Refer to a specialist if CKD stage G4 or 5, ACR >70, stage A2 plus haematuria, sustained decrease in GFR, poorly controlled hypertension despite at least 4 antihypertensive drugs or suspected renal artery stenosis.
- CKD monitoring should be at least annually in stages G1 to G3a, twice annually in stages G3b–G4 and 4 times a year in stage G5 kidney failure.
- Safety net – return if symptoms worsen and monitor U&Es.

Role play

Information for doctor	Additional information for role player
Patient: Mrs AB *Age*: 72 years *SH*: Lives with husband, retired. *PMH*: Type 2 diabetes *DH*: Gliclazide 80 mg OD *Information*: Had recent routine blood tests: • urea 18 mmol/l (NR: 4–6) • creatinine 260 mmol/l (NR: 64–111) • eGFR 28 ml/min/1.73 m^2 Last blood tests 6 months ago: • urea 12 mmol/l • creatinine 170 mmol/l. You are a GP Registrar.	*PC*: "*I was asked to come to discuss my blood test results*". *HPC*: Feels more tired than usual. No haematuria. No ankle oedema. No weight loss. No vomiting. Gets up 2 times at night to pass urine. *FH*: Nil *ICE*: Worried about her kidneys getting worse. *O/E*: BP 170/95. BMI 26. Slight pallor. Abdominal examination – NAD. No palpable kidneys or bladder.

ENT

Sore throat

- Very common presentation in general practice, and is usually caused by an infection in the throat.
- 50–70% of sore throats are viral (*SIGN*, 2010, *Guideline 117: Management of sore throat*).
- Tonsillitis is an infection of the tonsils at the back of the throat and symptoms are similar to a sore throat but may be more severe.
- The Centor clinical prediction score should be used to assist the decision on whether to prescribe an antibiotic.

Data gathering

Open question
- *"Can you tell me more about your sore throat?"*

Focused/closed questions

HPC: *"When did the sore throat first start?"*
"Have you also had a cough?" "If so, have you coughed up any phlegm?" "What colour?"
"Have you had a fever?"
"Have you had any pain when swallowing?" "Are you able to eat and drink ok?" (red flag if unable to swallow liquids)
"Have you had any diarrhoea or vomiting?"
"Have you had any aching muscles or excessive tiredness?
"Have you tried any treatments so far?"
"Is anyone else at home unwell?" "Have you been in contact with anyone else who is unwell?"
"Have you been abroad recently?" "If so, where?"

PMH: *"How is your health generally?" "Do you have any medical conditions?"*

DH: *"Do you take any regular medications?" "Have you taken any over-the-counter medicines?"*

SH: *"How is this sore throat affecting you in terms of school/work?"*

ICE: *"What prompted you to come in today?*

Examination:
- Temperature and pulse.
- Cervical lymph nodes.
- ENT examination – check throat and ears.
- Examination of chest.
- Abdominal examination to check for hepatosplenomegaly if suspecting glandular fever.

Clinical management

Investigations
- No specific investigations required unless suspecting glandular fever in which case a blood test should be done (FBC, CRP, LFTs, Paul Bunnell test).

Explanation to patient
- A sore throat is normally a symptom of a bacterial or viral infection, such as the common cold.
- Most sore throats are not serious and pass within a few days without the need for medical treatment. Over-the-counter painkillers, such as paracetamol or ibuprofen, can usually relieve the symptoms of a sore throat without the need to see a GP.

Management
- Watch and wait – many throat infections will resolve without any treatment.
- Salt water gargle.
- Simple analgesia, e.g. paracetamol, ibuprofen, Difflam spray.
- Encourage oral fluids.
- Antibiotics if suspecting bacterial tonsillitis.
- Refer to ENT urgently if suspecting quinsy (tonsillar abscess).
- Safety net – if stridor or acute respiratory distress refer immediately to hospital and don't examine throat.
- In cases of recurrent tonsillitis, consider tonsillectomy if >7 well documented and treated episodes of tonsillitis within 1 year, or ≥5 episodes in each of the previous 2 years, or ≥3 episodes in each of the previous 3 years.

Role play

Information for doctor	Additional information for role player
Patient: Miss ZA *Age:* 17 years *PMH:* Eczema *DH:* Cetraben BD, hydrocortisone 1% PRN. *Information:* You are a salaried GP and have a telephone consultation booked with this patient to discuss her sore throat.	*PC:* *"I have had a sore throat for 4 days now and it's not improving".* *HPC:* No cough or fever. Pain when swallowing – able to swallow liquids and solids, however. **No D&V. No tiredness. No foreign travel and no-one else unwell at home**. *SH:* Lives with parents. Smokes 5 cigs/day. *ICE:* Would like some antibiotics for her throat.

Labyrinthitis

- Condition due to inflammation of the labyrinth in the inner ear, although sometimes the vestibular nerve is also involved.
- Most commonly caused by a viral infection and typically causes vertigo and/or vomiting.
- Most cases ease within a few weeks.

Data gathering

Open question
- *"Can you describe the symptoms you have been experiencing?"*

Focused/closed questions

HPC: *"Have you been feeling dizzy?" "When did it first start?" "Have you experienced a spinning sensation with the dizziness?"*
"Have you had any nausea or vomiting?"
"Have you had any earache?"
"Have you had any problems with your hearing?"
"Have you had any ringing in your ears?" "Is the ringing in one ear?" (red flag)
"Have you had any numbness or weakness?"

PMH: *"Have you had a flu-like illness recently?" "Have you had any problems with your ears before?"*

DH: *"Do you take any regular medications?"* (beta blockers and aminoglycosides can cause vertigo)

SH: Drugs/alcohol/illicit drugs? *"Do you have stairs at home?" "Do you normally drive?" "Who lives with you at home?"*

ICE: *"Do you have any concerns about the dizziness, for example, falling at home?"*

Examination
- ENT exam.
- Neurological examination including cranial nerves and cerebellar signs.
- Hallpike manoeuvre.

Clinical management

Investigations
- Blood test – FBC, U&Es, TFTs, glucose.
- Audiometry.

Explanation to patient
- Labyrinthitis is an inner ear infection. It causes a delicate structure deep inside your ear, called the labyrinth, to become inflamed, affecting your hearing and balance.

Management

- Reassurance.
- Medication, e.g. stemetil or antihistamines.
- No driving.
- Refer urgently if suspected acoustic neuroma or if symptoms not improving by 6 weeks.

Role play

Information for doctor	Additional information for role player
Patient: Mrs EK *Age*: 80 years *PMH*: Atrial fibrillation, TIA 2008. *SH*: Lives alone in warden controlled flat. *DH*: Warfarin 5 mg OD. Simvastatin 40 mg OD. Bisoprolol 2.5 mg OD. *Information*: You are a GP registrar and have been asked to visit this patient today due to dizziness. You contact her by phone before visiting to clarify the reason for the visit.	*PC*: *"I have been feeling giddy since yesterday"* *HPC*: Constant dizziness and also spinning sensation. **Had flu 2 weeks ago. Nausea but no vomiting.** No earache or hearing loss. **No tinnitus**. *SH*: Doesn't drive. *ICE*: Worried about falling or going out as lives alone. Would like a visit as doesn't feel well enough to come to the surgery.

Hearing loss

- Can be classified as conductive, sensorineural or mixed hearing loss, and may be unilateral or bilateral.
- Can range from mild hearing impairment (27–40 decibels) to profound hearing impairment (>91 decibels).
- Rinne's and Weber's tests can be used to distinguish between conductive and sensorineural hearing loss.
- During the consultation you may have to write things down in order for the patient to understand, or alternatively they may be able to lip read.

Data gathering

Open question

- *"Can you tell me more about the hearing problems you have been experiencing?"*

Focused/closed questions

HPC: *"When did the hearing problem first start?"* *"Did it occur suddenly?"*
"Does it affect both ears?"
"What sounds are you able to hear, if any?"

"Have you noticed any ringing in your ears?" (red flag if unilateral)
"Any problem with your balance?" (red flag)
"Have you experienced any pain in your ears?"
"Do you suffer with any dizziness or vertigo?"
"Have you had any previous trauma or injury to your ears?"

PMH: Any previous problems with your ears, or any previous ear operations? Have you had many ear infections in the past? Any history of mumps or meningitis?

DH: Are you taking any regular medications? Have you taken gentamicin in the past?

FH: Is there a family history of hearing problems?

SH: Smoking/alcohol/illicit drug history? Occupation? Who lives with you at home?

ICE: *"Do you have any idea what might be causing the hearing loss?"*
"How has this hearing loss affected life at home and at work?"

Examination:
- Otoscopy.
- Whispered speech test.
- Rinne's and Weber's tests.

Clinical management

Investigations
- Audiometry.
- MRI of brain – if concerned about acoustic neuroma.

Explanation to patient
- Conductive deafness results from failure in any of the mechanisms that normally conduct sound waves through the outer ear, the eardrum or the bones of the middle ear.
- Sensorineural deafness results from a problem in the inner ear, especially the cochlea where sound vibrations are converted into nerve signals, or in any part of the brain that subsequently processes these signals.

Management
- Self help – ensure good lighting and sit close to the person you are talking to.
- Wax removal.
- Antibiotics if ear infection.
- Hearing aid or cochlear implants.
- Surgery – for some cases of perforated ear drum or for acoustic neuroma.
- Hearing dogs and assistive devices.
- Safety net – if problem worsening return to GP.
- Further details through Royal National Institute for Deaf People (www.rnid.org.uk)

Role play

Information for doctor	Additional information for role player
Patient: Mrs ED *Age*: 52 years *PMH*: Hysterectomy in 2005 *DH*: Nil *FH*: Nil *Information*: Last consultation was 4 months ago with GP Registrar – right acute otitis media. You are a salaried GP.	*PC*: Decreased hearing in right ear for past couple of months. *HPC*: **No pain in the ear. No tinnitus.** Gradual deterioration. No dizziness or balance problems. **No trauma.** *SH*: School teacher. **Lives alone.** No FH of hearing problems. *ICE*: Worried about going completely deaf. *O/E*: Decreased hearing on right side. Otoscopy NAD. Abnormal Rinne's test in right ear.

Tinnitus

- Symptom of abnormal noises, usually ringing or buzzing, heard inside the ear.
- The noise does not come from an external source.
- The cause is often not known, but can be a symptom of Ménière's disease or following a head injury or exposure to loud noise.
- Persistent unilateral tinnitus can be caused by an acoustic neuroma.
- There is no cure but there are various ways to reduce the symptoms.

Data gathering

Open questions

- *"Can you describe the noises in your ears that you've been experiencing?"*
- *"What do you mean by noises in your ears?"*

Focused/closed questions

HPC: *"When did the problem first start?"*
"What specific noises do you hear inside your ear?"
"Do you hear the noises all the time?"
"Do you hear the noises in both ears, or just one?" (red flag if unilateral)
"Are the noises coming from inside the ear or outside?"
"Have you experienced any other symptoms, for example visual changes, dizziness, headache or problems with balance?"
"Any history of injury to the ear or a head injury?" (red flag)
"Have you been exposed to loud noises recently?"
"Have you tried anything so far to get rid of the tinnitus?"
"Have you noticed any hearing loss? (possible Ménière's disease)
"Have you had any earache?"

PMH: Do you have any medical conditions? Any previous surgery?

DH: *"Are you on any regular medications?"* (e.g. aspirin, NSAIDs, frusemide and gentamicin can cause tinnitus)

SH: Smoking/alcohol/illicit drug history? Occupation? Who lives with you at home?

ICE: *"What were you hoping we could do to help?"*

"How has this been affecting you in terms of day to day life?" "Has it stopped you from doing anything you would usually be doing?"

Examination:
- BP.
- Otoscopy.
- Whispered speech test.
- Cranial nerve examination.
- Mental state examination – if need to rule out noises as being auditory hallucinations.

Clinical management

Investigations
- FBC (anaemia can cause tinnitus).
- Audiometry (if indicated).
- Brain MRI scan (if indicated).

Explanation to patient
- The ringing/buzzing noise inside your ear is called tinnitus.
- It is a fairly common problem and although there is no cure, there are various ways to make it more manageable.
- It is thought that signals are sent from the ear down the ear nerve to the hearing part of the brain where they are interpreted as noise.
- People often find that the noise is worse at night when you are in a quiet place.

Management
- Self help (see www.tinnitus.org.uk).
- Reassurance – most self resolve.
- If caused by a medication then stop this medication.
- SSRIs are sometimes used if associated anxiety and/or depression.
- 'Sound therapy' – having radio or TV on as background noise.
- Hearing aid – if hearing problem.
- Refer to tinnitus clinic.
- Refer to ENT urgently if any suspicion of acoustic neuroma.

Role play

Information for doctor	Additional information for role player
Patient: Mrs LW *Age*: 57 years *SH*: Lives with husband. Housewife. *FH*: Nil *PMH*: Dyspepsia *DH*: Omeprazole 40 mg daily. *Information*: No recent consultations. You are a salaried GP.	*PC*: "*I hear a ringing noise in my ears*". *HPC*: First started about 4 weeks ago. Ringing in both ears. **Noise from inside head. Worse at night. No earache. No visual symptoms or headache. No vomiting or dizziness. No trauma.** Exposure to loud noise at a concert prior to the ringing starting. *ICE*: Would like to know what is causing it and how to get rid of it. *O/E*: Hearing and otoscopy – NAD. Cranial nerves – NAD.

Obstructive sleep apnoea

- Condition in which there is intermittent and recurrent upper airway collapse during sleep.
- Periods of apnoea occur during sleep, when a patient stops breathing for 10 seconds or more.
- As a result of this disturbed sleep, patients often feel tired during the day.
- Most commonly occurs in middle aged, overweight males.
- Smoking, drinking alcohol in the evening, taking sedative drugs and enlarged tonsils are other risk factors.

Data gathering

Open question

- "*Could you tell me a bit more about the breathing problems you've been having at night?*"

Focused/closed questions

HPC: "*When did you first start experiencing these episodes?*"

"*How many episodes do you have in a typical night?*"

"*Has anyone witnessed these episodes?*" "*What exactly happens?*"

"*Do you feel tired during the day as a result?*"

"*Do you usually snore?*"

"*Do you have difficulty concentrating during the day?*"

"*Have you had any choking episodes during the night?*"

"*Has your partner ever mentioned that you are more irritable or restless at night?*"

PMH: Any previous medical problems or any previous ENT surgery?

DH: Do you take any regular medications? Any sleeping tablets?

SH: Smoking/alcohol/illicit drug history? Occupation? Who lives with you at home? Do you drive?

ICE: *"What specific concerns do you have about this sleep problem?"*

Examination:
- Weight/BMI.
- ENT examination – inspect tonsils and nasal passages.
- Neck circumference – <37 cm is low risk of OSA and >48 cm is high risk.

Clinical management

Investigations
- Epworth sleepiness scale.
- Refer for formal sleep study (polysomnography).

Explanation to patient
- Obstructive sleep apnoea syndrome is a condition where your breathing stops for short spells when you are asleep.
- It occurs because the throat muscles relax and become so floppy that they cause a temporary blockage of the airway. It usually wakes you up due to the decreased blood oxygen level and then when you start breathing again you will normally go off to sleep again.

Management
- General measures – weight loss if overweight, decrease alcohol intake and stop smoking, and sleep on side.
- Mandibular advancement device (dental appliance similar to a gum shield) for mild OSAS.
- Safety net – return if above measures not helping.
- CPAP for moderate to severe OSAS.
- Surgery – adeno-tonsillectomy if large tonsils or adenoids.
- DVLA – must inform DVLA and must not drive until satisfactory control of symptoms.

Role play

Information for doctor	Additional information for role player
Patient: Mr JH *Age*: 62 years *SH*: Unemployed, lives with wife *PMH*: COPD, obesity *DH*: Seretide 500 mcg BD, spiriva 18 mcg 2 puffs OD, salbutamol 2 puffs PRN. *Information*: Last seen 1 month ago for COPD review. You are a salaried GP.	*PC*: *"My wife is concerned about my snoring".* *HPC*: *"She also said that I stop breathing in the night periodically".* 2–3 episodes per night. Started approx 2 months ago. **Tiredness during the day and poor concentration.** *"Wife also thinks I'm more irritable".* *SH*: Smokes 20 cigs/day. Alcohol 40 units/week. *ICE*: **Would like something to stop the snoring.** *O/E*: Weight 110 kg (BMI 37), throat – NAD. Large nasal polyp visualised in left nostril.

Ophthalmology

Red eye

- Red eye is a relatively common presentation in primary care, most of which are due to quite trivial causes.
- Causes of painful red eye include acute angle closure glaucoma, keratitis, trauma and acute anterior uveitis.
- Causes of painless red eye include conjunctivitis, episcleritis and subconjunctival haemorrhage.

Data gathering

Open question
- *"Can you tell me more about your eye symptoms?"*

Focused/closed questions
HPC: *"When did the problem first start?"*
"Have your symptoms got worse since then?"
"Is the eye painful? If so, how severe?" (red flag if severe pain)
"Is your vision affected?"
"Did you get a sudden loss of vision?" (red flag)
"Any watering or itchiness of the eye?"
"Have you experienced any discharge from your eyes?"
"Any trauma or contact with chemicals in the eye?" (red flag)
"Have you noticed that your eye is more sensitive to the light?"
"Have you had any floaters or flashing lights in your field of vision?
"Have you suffered from any headache, vomiting, rash, fever?" (red flags)
"Any contact with other people with red/sticky eyes?"
"Do you wear contact lenses?"
"Have you had a recent cold or viral infection?"

PMH: Do you have any medical conditions, e.g. diabetes?
Any previous eye problems or eye surgery?

SH: Smoking/alcohol/illicit drug history? Occupation? Exposure to chemicals?

FH: Any FH of eye problems?

ICE: *"Do you have any idea what might be causing these eye problems?"*

Examination:
- Inspection of the eye including sclera and lids (can use fluoroscein drops).
- Visual acuity, visual fields and eye movements.
- Pupil reflexes.
- Systems examination if suspecting systemic cause.
- Palpation of the temporal area (if suspecting temporal arteritis).

Clinical management

Investigations
- Slit lamp examination.

Explanation to patient
- There are numerous different causes of red eye, which can be categorised into painful and painless.
- The commonest cause is conjunctivitis which is redness and inflammation of the thin layer of tissue that covers the front of the eye (conjunctiva). This results from a bacterial or viral infection or from an allergic reaction.
- Some cases of red eye require urgent treatment, and it is therefore important to be able to distinguish between the different causes.

Management
- Same day ophthalmology referral if moderate to severe eye pain, reduced visual acuity, unilateral red eye, abnormal pupillary reactions or suspected penetrating trauma injury.
- Safety net – in all other cases if no improvement in symptoms over the next few days return to the GP.

Acute painful red eye
- Acute angle closure glaucoma (severe pain, haloes around lights, vomiting). Signs include decreased visual acuity, hazy cornea, fixed semi-dilated pupil. Refer immediately.
- Acute anterior uveitis (photophobia, blurred vision, headache). Signs include decreased visual acuity, red eye, constricted or irregular pupil. Refer within 24 hours.
- Trauma to eye – painful eye. Refer immediately if risk of serious trauma.

Acute non-painful red eye
- Conjunctivitis (mild discomfort, discharge from eye). Signs include normal visual acuity and unilateral or bilateral discharge. Treat with chloramphenicol or sodium cromoglycate.
- Subconjunctival haemorrhage (spontaneous or traumatic). Signs include normal visual acuity with blood under conjunctiva. Usually self resolving. Check BP.

Role play

Information for doctor	Additional information for role player
Patient: Mr GR *Age*: 36 years *SH*: Lives with wife and 3 children. Builder. *PMH*: Crohn's disease *DH*: Azathioprine 75 mg OD *Information*: Called the surgery this morning requesting an urgent appointment due to eye symptoms. You are a GP Partner.	*PC*: *"I've got a pain in my right eye".* *HPC*: Pain started last night but not worsening. **Constant moderate pain**. Also red eye. No trauma. No fever. Vision decreased in right eye. **Photophobia.** No headache or vomiting. **Watering of eye but no itchiness. Doesn't wear contact lenses. No exposure to chemicals.** *FH*: **Nil** *ICE*: Worried about going blind. *O/E*: BP 130/60. Injection around the right iris and photophobia in the right eye when a direct light is shone. Fundoscopy NAD.

Neurology

Headache

- The 2012 NICE guidelines (*CG150: Headaches*) define headaches as follows:
  - Primary headache disorders: not associated with underlying pathology, e.g. tension headache, cluster headaches, migraines.
  - Secondary headache disorders: headache attributed to underlying pathology, e.g. from infection, neoplasm or associated with medication overuse.
- Chronic headache is defined as headaches for over 15 days per month for more than 3 months.
- The commonest type of headache seen in primary care is a tension-type headache.

Data gathering

Open question
- *"Can you tell me more about your headache?"*

Focused/closed questions

HPC: *"Where exactly are you experiencing the pain?"* *"Does the pain spread anywhere else?"*
"When did it first start? Is it a constant or intermittent pain?"
"How frequently are you getting headaches?"
"How severe is the pain?"
"Is the headache getting worse?" (red flag)
"Any nausea, vomiting, fever, neck stiffness, visual symptoms or rash?" (red flags)
"Is it worse at any particular time of the day?" (worse in morning if raised ICP)
"Was the headache of sudden onset?" (red flag)
"Have you had any seizures or noticed any personality changes?" (red flags)
"Have you suffered from a head injury recently?" (red flag)

PMH: Any past history of migraines/ headaches?

DH: *"Do you take any regular medications?"* Codeine?

FH: Any family history of migraine?

SH: Smoking/alcohol/illicit drug history? Occupation? Stress? Who lives with you at home?

ICE: *"What worries you about this headache?"*
"How is this headache affecting your daily activities?"
Examination: • BP.
• Neurological examination including cranial nerves.
• Fundoscopy.
• Palpation of temporal arteries.

Clinical management

Investigations
• Not routinely required.
• Brain MRI if suspected brain pathology.

Explanation to patient
• Tension headaches – typically the pain is around the 'hat-band' area. Can be described as a squeezing or pressure on the head. Usually on both sides of the head, and usually lasts a few hours. Often caused by stress or physical tension.
• Cluster headaches – pain typically lasts 45–90 minutes and attacks usually occur one to two times daily. The clusters of headaches usually last from a few weeks to a few months. The pain is centred around or behind the eye, temple or forehead and is unilateral. The pain is often accompanied by watering of the eye on the same side, runny nose or nasal congestion.

Management
(based on *SIGN*, 2008, *Guideline 107: Diagnosis and management of headaches in adults* and *NICE,* 2012, *CG150: Headaches*)
• Headache diary.
• Tension headache: exercise, paracetamol, NSAIDs, and eliminate stressors. Consider a course of 10 sessions of acupuncture for the prophylactic treatment of tension headaches.
• Cluster headache: oxygen and sumatriptan for an acute attack. Consider verapamil for prophylactic treatment during a bout of cluster headaches.
• Migraine – see next topic.
• Safety net – if not improving to return to GP.
• Headache 'red flags' to trigger referral include sudden onset headache reaching maximum intensity within 5 minutes, headache associated with new onset neurological, cognitive or personality change, recent head trauma within 3 months or symptoms suggestive of giant cell arteritis or acute glaucoma.

Role play

Information for doctor	Additional information for role player
Patient: Mr BA *Age*: 28 years *SH*: Investment banker *FH*: Nil *PMH*: Nil *DH*: Nil *Information*: Recent consultation with locum GP due to headaches. Neurological examination – NAD. You are a GP Partner.	*PC*: "*I saw one of the other doctors recently due to headaches but they're not getting any better*." *HPC*: Headaches occurring every day for past 2 weeks. Headaches come and go (approx 2× daily). Pain mainly across forehead. No visual symptoms. No nausea, vomiting, fever or neck stiffness. Has been very busy at work and under quite a lot of stress. Recently broke up with girlfriend. *ICE*: Would like some painkillers for the headache as paracetamol and ibuprofen not helping. *O/E*: BP 110/70. Fundoscopy – NAD.

Migraine

- A condition causing severe headache often with associated nausea, vomiting or visual symptoms.
- Between migraine attacks the symptoms completely resolve.
- The two main types of migraine are classic migraine (migraine with aura) and common migraine (migraine without aura).

Data gathering

Open question
- "*Can you tell me more about your headache?*"

Focused/closed questions
HPC: "*Where exactly is the location of the pain?*"

"*Do you get any associated nausea or vomiting with the headache?*"

"*Is the headache worse at any particular time of the day?*"

"*Do you get any visual symptoms or pins and needles associated with the headache?*"

"*Are your eyes more sensitive to bright lights?*"

"*Have you noticed any muscle weakness or altered sensation?*"

"*Is there any warning prior to the onset of the headache?*"

"*Are there any particular triggers or any aggravating factors?*" (e.g. caffeine, chocolate, red wine)

"*Any relieving factors?*"

"*Have you noticed any problems with your balance or co-ordination?*" (possible red flag)

"*Have you noticed any change in your headaches depending on your menstrual cycle?*"

PMH: *"Have you suffered from migraines in the past?"*
DH: Are you on any regular medications? Do you take the combined contraceptive pill? (contraindicated if migraine with aura).
FH: Any FH of headaches/migraines?
SH: Smoking/alcohol/illicit drug history? Occupation? Stress?
ICE: "Do you have any thoughts as to what is causing these headaches?"
Examination:
- BP.
- Neurological examination including cranial nerves.
- Fundoscopy.

Clinical management

Investigations

- No specific investigations (clinical diagnosis).
- Only if ruling out other causes of headaches, e.g. CT brain to rule out intracranial bleed or tumour.

Explanation to patient

- The pain of a migraine occurs when excited nerve cells trigger a nerve in the head to release chemicals that irritate and cause swelling of the blood vessels on the surface of the brain. These swollen vessels then send pain signals to an area of the brain that processes pain information.
- There are two types of migraine – a classical migraine which is when you have a warning sign, known as an aura, before the migraine begins, and a common migraine when there is no warning sign.
- A class of drugs called triptans are used to treat migraines. They cause the blood vessels around the brain to constrict. This reverses the widening of blood vessels which is believed to be part of the migraine process.

Management

(based on *NICE*, 2012, *CG150: Headaches*)

- Acute treatment – offer a combination of triptans and NSAIDs or paracetamol. Do not use opioids.
- Prophylaxis – offer topiramate or propranolol and avoid triggers.
- Menstrual migraine – offer triptans e.g. zolmitriptan 2.5 mg BD on the days migraine is expected.
- Second line treatments include gabapentin or acupuncture.
- Consider an anti-emetic in addition to acute treatment even in the absence of nausea and vomiting.
- Advise patients that riboflavin (vitamin B_2) 400mg daily may be effective in reducing migraine frequency and intensity.
- Safety net – refer if uncertain diagnosis or not controlled with above treatments.

Role play

Information for doctor	Additional information for role player
Patient: Ms JB *Age*: 25 years *SH*: Lives with friends. Postgraduate student. Alcohol 6 units/week. *FH*: Nil *PMH*: Nil *DH*: Microgynon *Information*: You are a GP Registrar.	*PC*: *"I've recently been getting very bad headaches".* *HPC*: Three episodes of bad headaches in the past month. Last for approx. 1 day. Pain on left side of head. **Also had some numbness of the face prior to the headache. No visual symptoms except photophobia.** No vomiting but nausea. Paracetamol not helping. **No known food triggers – rarely drinks red wine or caffeinated drinks.** *ICE*: **Worried it may be related to the contraceptive pill.** *O/E*: Neurological exam – NAD, fundoscopy – NAD.

Collapse and seizures

Data gathering

Open question

- *"Can you describe what happened?"*

Focused/closed questions

HPC: *"How did you feel beforehand?" "Did you get any warning before it happened?"*
"Did you have any chest pain/palpitations/dizziness?"
"Were there any triggers for the collapse?"
"Did anyone witness the collapse/seizure?" "Did you lose consciousness?"
"Did you lose control of your bladder?" "Did you bite your tongue?"
"Did you have any jerking of your limbs?" "Was it a first seizure?" (red flag)
"Did you injure yourself?"
"How did you feel afterwards? "Did you feel drowsy afterwards?"

PMH: *"Any previous seizures or history of epilepsy?"*

DH: *"Do you take any regular medications?"* (e.g. beta blockers, tricyclic antidepressants and amiodarone could all cause collapse)

SH: *"Do you normally drive?"* Occupation? Alcohol/smoking/illicit drug history?

FH: *"Any history of heart disease or sudden death?"*

ICE: *"What do you think caused the collapse?"*

Examination: • BP (lying and standing); pulse.
• Cardiovascular examination.
• Neurological examination.

Clinical management

Investigations
- Blood test – FBC, U&Es, TFTs, glucose.
- ECG.

Explanation to patient
- A seizure is an episode caused by a burst of abnormal electrical activity in the brain. Typically, a seizure lasts from a few seconds to a few minutes.
- There are different types of seizures, broadly classified into two types – generalized seizures and partial seizures.
- Generalised seizures occur if you have a burst of abnormal electrical activity which affects the whole of the brain, whereas partial seizures only affect one part of the brain, resulting in localised (focal) symptoms.
- Alternatively, a collapse may be due to a blackout which describes a loss of vision and momentary lapse of consciousness due to diminished circulation to the brain.

Management
- If suspected seizure, refer to neurology/first seizure clinic.
- If recurrent blackouts also refer to neurology.
- Inform DVLA (see *Appendix 4*).

Role play

Information for doctor	Additional information for role player
Patient: Mr TA *Age*: 37 years *PMH*: Migraine *SH*: Lives with wife and 2 children. HGV driver. Drinks 30 units alcohol/week. No illicit drug use. *DH*: Sumatriptan s/c 4 mg PRN. *Information*: You are a locum GP. This patient has an emergency appointment with you today. He was last seen 6 months ago due to migraines.	*PC*: *"I think I might have had a fit last night"* *HPC*: Returned from work yesterday and shortly afterwards had a funny turn witnessed by his daughter. She described him being unresponsive for a few seconds with shaking of arms and legs. **No tongue biting or urinary incontinente. Felt tired afterwards.** Went to A&E but long wait and better by then. Didn't feel unwell beforehand. **No head injury or trauma. First episode**. *FH*: No FH of epilepsy, neurological conditions or sudden death. *ICE*: Worried that it might happen again. *O/E*: BP 100/60. HR 50, regular. HS I + II +0. Neuro exam – NAD.

Multiple sclerosis

- MS is a disorder of the central nervous system resulting in damage to the nerve fibres that carry messages to and from the brain.
- Symptoms can occur in any part of the body, and include numbness, tingling, blurring of vision, muscle weakness and problems with mobility/balance.
- Symptoms can initially come and go, and then usually with time become permanent.
- Thought to be an auto-immune cause, resulting in inflammation of the myelin sheath around the nerve fibre.
- There are three main types – relapsing remitting, primary progressive or secondary progressive.
- There is increasing evidence that early diagnosis and treatment may delay, or even prevent, the previously inevitable disability.

Data gathering

Open question
- *"Can you tell me what symptoms have you been experiencing?"*

Focused/closed questions
HPC: *"When did these symptoms first start?"*
"Have you experienced any weakness/numbness/balance problems/ visual symptoms?"
"Have you experienced any pain?" "If so, what type of pain is it?"
"Have you had any problems with your speech or swallowing?"
"Have you had any problems with your memory or concentration?"
"Have you had any problems with controlling your bowels or bladder?"
"Have you had any problems with muscle spasms or mobility?"
"Are these symptoms constant or intermittent?" "Are they worsening?"
"Have you felt more tired than usual?"
PMH: Any history of any medical conditions?
FH: Any family history of neurological problems or MS?
DH: Do you take any regular medications?
SH: Who lives with you at home? Smoking/alcohol/illicit drug history? Occupation?
ICE: *"How are you managing at home with these symptoms?"*
Examination: • Neurological examination including cranial nerves
- Eye examination

Clinical management

Investigations
- MRI of brain.
- Blood tests – FBC, ESR, CRP, U&Es, LFTs, calcium, glucose, thyroid, B_{12}, HIV serology.

- Visual evoked potential studies.
- Lumbar puncture.

Explanation to patient

- Multiple sclerosis (MS) is a disease of the central nervous system (brain and spinal cord). White matter within the brain or spinal cord becomes inflamed and is then destroyed by the person's own immune system. These inflamed areas become scarred, giving the disease its name: multiple areas of hardening (sclerosis) within the brain or spinal cord.

Management

(based on *NICE, 2014, CG186: Multiple sclerosis*)

- If suspected MS refer to neurology for confirmatory diagnosis.
- For acute episodes with disabling symptoms – high dose methylprednisolone for 3–5 days. Also, refer to a specialist neurological rehabilitation service.
- Immunomodulatory agents, e.g. beta-interferon – can reduce the number of relapses.
- Other medications for specific symptoms, e.g. anti-spasmodics, anti-depressants and anti-cholinergics. Offer amantadine to treat fatigue and prompt treatment with antibiotics if UTI.
- Physiotherapy, occupational therapy, speech therapy, psychological therapy.
- Safety net – return to GP if symptoms not improving within 1–2 weeks.

Role play

Information for doctor	Additional information for role player
Patient: Ms SC *Age*: 37 years *SH*: Lives alone. Receptionist. *PMH*: Polycystic ovarian syndrome *DH*: Nil *Information*: No recent consultations. You are a salaried GP.	*PC*: *"I seem to be more unsteady on my feet, and fell over yesterday".* *HPC*: 4-week history of problems with balance. Not improving. **Also blurring of vision in left eye and pain behind left eye.** No earache. No headache. No numbness but muscle weakness in both legs. **No bowel or bladder symptoms. No speech problems. Poor concentration and memory not as good. General lethargy.** *FH*: Nil *ICE*: Worried about a brain tumour. *O/E*: Fundoscopy – blurring of left optic disc. Neurological examination – decreased sensation in left leg. Power decreased in lower limbs bilaterally.

Parkinson's disease

- A progressive neurological condition where cells in a section of the brain called the substantia nigra degenerate.
- Symptoms include tremor, rigidity and bradykinesia.
- It mainly affects people over the age of 50 and is more common with increasing age.

Data gathering

Open question

- *"Can you tell me more about your problems with walking?"*

Focused/closed questions

HPC: *"Have you had any muscle stiffness or tremor?"*
"Have you noticed any change to your walking?"
"Have you noticed any changes to your handwriting?"
"Have you had more difficulties with tasks such as tying shoe laces and buttoning shirts?"
"Have you had any problems with your balance?"
"Have you been falling more than usual?"
"Have you had any problems with your speech?"
"Have you been feeling low in mood?" (red flag)
"Have you been incontinent of urine?" (red flag)

DH: *"Do you take any regular medications"* (phenothiazines and haloperidol can cause Parkinsonian symptoms)

SH: *"Who lives with you at home?" "What support network do you have?"*
"What is your occupation?" "Do you normally drive?"

ICE: *"What concerns you about your symptoms?"*

Examination:
- Inspection – features include expressionless face, drooling, pill-rolling tremor.
- Speech – reduced volume and monotonous tone.
- Neurological examination – cogwheel rigidity. Normal power and reflexes.
- Gait – shuffling gait with reduced arm swing, slowness of movements, difficulty initiating walking.
- Handwriting – micrographia.
- Glabellar tap – tap the patient on their forehead and they will continue to blink if Parkinson's disease (PD).

Clinical management

Investigations

- No specific investigations for PD – diagnosis based on history.

Explanation to patient

- PD is a condition affecting the way the brain coordinates the movements of the muscles in various parts of the body.
- The three main symptoms are slowness of movement, shaking and muscle stiffness.

Management

- There is no cure – treatment only relieves symptoms.
- Refer to neurology for initial assessment and treatment.
- Consider referral for physiotherapy, OT, speech therapy, specialist nurse and dietitian. T'ai chi is effective in improving stability and balance.
- Medication for treatment of motor symptoms – mild potency drugs include selegiline and amantadine. Moderate potency drugs include dopamine agonists, e.g. ropinirole. High potency drugs include levodopa.
- Medication for non-motor symptoms – pramipexole and venlafaxine are recommended for depression, melatonin can possibly be useful for insomnia and rivastigmine can be highly effective for dementia.
- Inform DVLA.
- Surgery – e.g. chronic deep brain stimulation to ease symptoms in severe cases.

Role play

Information for doctor	Additional information for role player
Patient: Mr KZ *Age*: 80 years *SH*: Retired builder. Lives with daughter. Never smoked. 2 units alcohol/week. *FH*: Both parents had strokes. *PMH*: Osteoarthritis right hip and both knees. Hypercholesterolaemia. *DH*: Naproxen 500 mg BD. Simvastatin 40 mg nocte. *Information*: You are a GP partner and have seen this patient on several occasions before.	*PC*: Daughter concerned about his mobility. *HPC*: Daughter worried as becoming more unsteady on his feet. Shuffling more when walking and has difficulty turning. Has tripped on a few occasions. **Also appears very shaky. Has difficulty dressing in the morning, but his daughter hasn't noticed problems with his handwriting. Also has muscle stiffness.** Not talking as much and daughter feels he is a bit down. *ICE*: Patient says he feels fine although acknowledges feeling unsteady on his feet. *O/E*: Expressionless face. Cogwheel rigidity. Shuffling gait. Stooped posture. Slow movements.

Temporal arteritis

- Condition of unknown aetiology, causing inflammation of the large and medium arteries of the head, most commonly the temporal artery.
- It is an uncommon condition, mainly affecting people over the age of 60.

- Can lead to serious conditions such as blindness and stroke.
- Symptoms include headache, jaw pain, scalp tenderness and visual disturbances.
- Up to half of people with temporal arteritis will develop a related condition called polymyalgia rheumatica (PMR).

Data gathering

Open question
- *"Can you tell me more about the symptoms you've been experiencing?"*

Focused/closed questions
HPC: *"When did these symptoms first start?"*
"Have your symptoms worsened since then?"
"Was it a sudden onset?"
"Have you experienced any headache, jaw pain, numbness or visual disturbances?"
"Have you had any scalp pain?"
"Do you have any tiredness or muscle weakness?"
"Have you had a fever, weight loss or loss of appetite?" (systemic symptoms)

PMH: *"Do you have any medical conditions?"*
DH: *"Do you take any regular medications?"*
SH: Who lives with you at home? Smoking/alcohol history?
ICE: *"What were you hoping we could do to help?"*

Examination:
- Palpation of head – prominence of temporal artery, tenderness +/– pulsation.
- Cranial nerve examination – including visual acuity and visual fields.
- Fundoscopy – pale swollen optic disc with possible haemorrhages.

Clinical management

Investigations
- Blood test – ESR.
- Temporal artery biopsy.

Explanation to patient
- Condition caused by inflammation of the arteries on the side of the head.

Management
- Refer to secondary care if temporal arteritis is suspected.
- High dose steroids (40–60 mg prednisolone, tapering down over several months).
- Low dose aspirin (75 mg).
- Safety net – if symptoms not improving return to GP.

Role play

Information for doctor	Additional information for role player
Patient: Mr GA *Age*: 63 years *SH*: Lives with wife. Retired. *FH*: Nil *DH*: Nil *PMH*: Bowel cancer in 2007. Had subtotal colectomy. *Information*: You are a GP Registrar	*PC*: "*I've been experiencing sharp pains around my eyes*". *HPC*: Started this morning. Normal visual acuity. Shooting pains around temples. **Very sensitive to touch. No muscle weakness or lethargy**. No jaw pain. **No fever, weight loss or loss of appetite.** *ICE*: Very worried at what is causing it. *O/E*: Temporal artery tenderness. Normal visual acuity. Fundoscopy normal.

Transient ischaemic attack

- Temporary lack of blood supply to the brain, resulting in symptoms similar to a stroke, but which resolve within 24 hours.
- Most commonly caused by a small blood clot, and is sometimes referred to as a 'mini stroke'.
- Treatment includes reducing any risk factors for developing a stroke, and medication to reduce the risk of blood clotting.

Data gathering

Open question
- "*Can you tell me more about the symptoms you have been experiencing?*"

Focused/closed questions
HPC: "*Have you experienced any weakness of your face, arms or legs? If so, which side is affected?*"

"*Do you have any problems with your speech, swallowing or vision?*"

"*Any numbness or pins and needles in any part of your body?*"

"*Has anyone else witnessed these changes?*"

"*Have the symptoms improved since they first started?*" "*If so, did the symptoms resolve within 24 hours?*" (red flag if residual focal neurology)

"*Have you had any dizziness, headache or loss of balance?*"

"*Have you had any loss of consciousness, confusion or seizures?*" (red flags)

PMH: Any previous history of TIA, stroke or heart problems? Any previous heart operations? Do you have high blood pressure or diabetes? (risk factors)

DH: Do you take any regular medications?

FH: Do you have any family history of diabetes, heart disease or stroke?

SH: Who lives with you at home? Support? Smoking/alcohol/illicit drug history? Occupation? Do you normally drive?

ICE: *"Do you have any ideas as to what is causing your symptoms?"*

Examination:
- BP and pulse (rate and rhythm).
- Cardiovascular system – check for heart murmurs and carotid bruits.
- Neurological examination and cranial nerves: check for weakness, visual loss and gait.

Clinical management

Investigations

- ECG – to check for atrial fibrillation.
- Use the Rosier Stroke Recognition score (www.derbygpvts.co.uk/lib/ROSIERv15.pdf)
- Blood test – FBC, fasting glucose, cholesterol (to check for risk factors), U&Es, LFTs, TFTs.
- Coagulation studies – may be required, but should be discussed with a specialist first.
- Echocardiogram – if suspecting cardiac valve problem.
- Doppler ultrasound scan of carotids, or MRI/CT brain – only if requested by a specialist.

Explanation to patient

- A TIA produces a group of symptoms which occur due to a temporary lack of blood to part of the brain. This usually happens due to a tiny blood clot blocking a small blood vessel in the brain, stopping the blood flow and starving part of the brain of oxygen. It usually only blocks the blood flow for a few minutes and then recovers back to normal. It is considered as a 'warning sign' that you are at higher risk of having a stroke or heart attack.
- You are at higher risk of a TIA or a stroke if you are overweight, smoke, have high blood pressure, high cholesterol or diabetes.

Management

(based on *NICE*, 2008, *CG68: Stroke*)

- In people with sudden onset of neurological symptoms, a validated tool such as FAST (face, arm, speech test) should be used to screen for the diagnosis of a stroke or TIA.
- People with a suspected TIA who are at high risk of a stroke (e.g. an $ABCD^2$ score* of 4 or above) should receive immediate aspirin 300 mg daily, specialist assessment within 24 hours of the onset of symptoms, and commencement of secondary prevention as soon as the diagnosis is confirmed.
- People with an ABCD2 score of 3 or below should have aspirin 300 mg daily started immediately and a specialist assessment as soon as possible but definitely within 1 week.

- Aspirin 300 mg should be commenced for at least 14 days (if no possibility of an intracranial bleed) followed by low dose aspirin (75 mg) together with dipyridamole.
- Reduce any risk factors, e.g. stop smoking, control high blood pressure, treat high cholesterol (consider atorvastatin 80 mg) and atrial fibrillation, weight loss and exercise.
- Patients with more than one TIA in a week should be investigated in hospital immediately, otherwise all patients should be seen in a TIA clinic within 1 week.
- Inform DVLA – patient must not drive for 1 month.
- Safety net – routinely review in the GP surgery within 1 week even if all the TIA symptoms have now resolved.

*ABCD^2 – scoring system to assess for high risk TIAs, taking into account **a**ge, **b**lood pressure, **c**linical features, **d**uration of symptoms and whether the patient is **d**iabetic (see *NICE*, 2008, *CG68: Stroke*).

Role play

Information for doctor	Additional information for role player
Patient: Mrs FY *Age*: 74 years old *SH*: Retired, lives with husband *PMH*: NIDDM *DH*: Metformin 850 mg TDS *Information*: Last consultation 2 weeks ago with practice nurse – BP 180/98 mmHg, BMI 34. You are a GP Registrar.	*PC*: Woke up this morning with slurred speech and weakness of left arm which has now resolved. **No visual symptoms. No headache or dizziness. Had problems with balance but now resolved.** No LOC or seizures. **Last cholesterol check was high (6.5) and has been trying to improve this through diet as not keen to take statins.** *ICE*: Concerned about a stroke as her husband had a stroke a few years ago. *O/E*: Neuro exam – NAD. Heart rate regular. BP 170/95.

Rheumatology and musculoskeletal

Back pain

- About 80% of people will have at least one bout of back pain in their lifetime.
- 'Non-specific' back pain is the most common type.
- Other causes of back pain include sciatica, cauda equina syndrome, ankylosing spondylitis and arthritis.

Data gathering

Open question
- *"Can you tell me more about the back pain you have been experiencing?"*

Focused/closed questions

HPC: *"When did the pain first start?" "Was there any injury or trauma?"*
"Where is the pain?" "Does the pain radiate anywhere else?"
"Is the pain constant?"
"Is the pain worse at any particular time of the day or night?" (red flag if night pain)
"What type of pain is it?"
"Are you able to walk?"
"Have you been experiencing any numbness or tingling of the legs or around the back passage?" (red flag)
"Have you ever lost control of your bowels or bladder?" (red flag)
"Any fever or weight loss?" (red flag)

PMH: Any history of back problems?

FH: Any family history of back problems?

DH: Are you taking any medications at present?

SH: Occupation? *"Does your job involve heavy lifting?" "Who lives with you at home?"*

ICE: *"How has this pain been affecting you at home and at work?"*

Examination:
- Back examination including straight leg raise and gait (see *Appendix 1*).
- Sensation and reflexes.

Clinical management

Investigations

- No investigations required for non-specific back pain.
- Bloods – ESR, bone profile, PSA (to rule out conditions such as ankylosing spondylitis or metastatic prostate cancer).
- Lumbo-sacral spinal X-ray – not routinely offered but can help to rule out conditions such as ankylosing spondylitis, vertebral collapse or cancer.
- MRI if considering other causes or possible surgery.

Explanation to patient

- Non-specific low back pain means that the pain is not due to any specific cause or underlying disease that can be found.
- In some cases the cause may be a sprain of a ligament or muscle, or a minor problem with a disc between two vertebrae (back bones).

Management

If back pain <6 weeks duration:

- Assess risk for chronicity using the START Back Screening Tool (http://patient.info/health/start-back-screening-tool-for-low-back-pain) – score <3 = low risk; score ≥4 = medium or high risk, depending on their psychiatry score.
- Exercise.
- Analgesia – paracetamol +/- NSAIDs, increasing to codeine or tramadol if required.
- Muscle relaxant – consider diazepam for short term use.
- Social – sick note, driving.
- Refer immediately if any signs of cauda equina syndrome.
- Routine referral if no improvement in 6 weeks.
- Safety net – return if not improving.

NICE recommendations

(2009, *CG88: Low back pain*) *for chronic non-specific back pain (lasting >6 weeks):*
- Tricyclic antidepressants, e.g. amitriptyline, if simple analgesics insufficient.
- Structured exercise programme.
- Manual therapy – physiotherapy, osteopath (several sessions of massage, spinal mobilisation and/or spinal manipulation). Consider Alexander technique (*BMJ*, 2008; 337: a884).
- Also consider acupuncture, CBT and/or referral to a pain clinic.

Role play

Information for doctor	Additional information for role player
Patient: Mr AK *Age*: 58 years *SH*: Lives with wife, works as builder *PMH*: Epilepsy *DH*: Phenytoin 300 mg OD *Information*: You are a GP Partner.	*PC*: "I've got really bad lower back pain". *HPC*: Back pain for 1 week. Slipped on concrete at work. **No radiation of pain down legs. No numbness/ tingling in legs. No urinary/bowel symptoms.** Pain constant but worse when moving. **Has tried ibuprofen so far and not helping much.** *ICE*: Would like an X-ray of his back and painkillers. *O/E*: Tenderness on flexion of back. Straight leg raise >50°, reflexes and sensation normal.

Shoulder pain

- The most common causes of shoulder pain seen in primary care are frozen shoulder, rotator cuff disorders, osteoarthritis and shoulder instability.
- Frozen shoulder (adhesive capsulitis) occurs when there is thickening, swelling and tightening of the tissues surrounding the shoulder joint. This results in decreased movement of the shoulder.
- The rotator cuff is a group of muscles around the shoulder joint which provides stability and movement of the shoulder. The rotator cuff can be affected by a tear, tendonitis or bursitis.
- Shoulder pain can also be caused by extrinsic causes, for example, polymyalgia rheumatica or referred pain from other structures such as the neck, heart or gallbladder.

Data gathering

Open question
- *"Can you tell me more about your shoulder pain?"*

Focused/closed questions

HPC: *"When did the pain first start?"*
"Which shoulder is affected?" "Are you left/right handed?"
"Did you injure your shoulder?" (red flag if unreduced dislocation)
"Where exactly is the pain?" "Does the pain spread anywhere?"
"Do you have decreased movement in the shoulder?"
"Do you get any pain at night?" (red flag)
"Do you have pain at rest or only on movement?"
"Does the pain restrict activities?"
"Do you have any pain in your neck?"
"Have you noticed any weight loss, lumps or swelling?" "Any fever or redness over the shoulder?" "Any numbness?" (red flags)

PMH: Any previous shoulder problems, or past surgery?
Any history of diabetes, cancer or ischaemic heart disease?

DH: *"Do you take any regular medications?"*

SH: Who lives with you at home? How are you coping at home? Occupation? Do you drive? Do you play any regular sports?

ICE: *"What were you expecting in terms of treatment for your shoulder problem?"*

Examination: • Shoulder examination (see *Appendix 1*).

Clinical management

Investigations
- Shoulder X-ray – if suspected bony injury.

- Shoulder MRI – if suspecting rotator cuff/soft tissue problem.
- Shoulder arthroscopy.
- Blood test – FBC, ESR, CRP (if red flag symptoms).

Explanation to patient

The commonest causes of shoulder pain are described below:

Common causes of shoulder pain	*Description*	*History*	*Examination*	*Explanation to patient*	*Management*
Rotator cuff tendinopathy	Degenerative changes of the tendons around the shoulder joint. Commonest cause of shoulder pain.	History of repetitive movement or heavy lifting.	Painful arc 60–120°. Pain on active/resisted movement; impingement.	Damage to the tissues that connect the muscles to bones at the shoulder joint.	Activity modification. Analgesia/NSAIDs, steroid injections, physiotherapy, surgery.
Rotator cuff tear	The rotator cuff is a group of four muscles and their tendons, providing shoulder stability. A tear is usually due to trauma. Most common in >40 age group.	Pain and weakness of shoulder.	Shoulder weakness. Unable to raise arm over head.	Tear to one or more of the four tendons of the rotator cuff muscles.	Analgesia, rest, orthopaedic referral for acute tear.
Adhesive capsulitis	Otherwise known as frozen shoulder. Can take up to 3 years to resolve. More common in 40–60 year age group and in diabetics.	Restricted shoulder movement and stiffness. Pain deep in joint.	Tenderness on palpation of shoulder joint. Decreased ROM of shoulder.	The tissues surrounding the shoulder joint become inflamed and stiff, restricting shoulder movement.	Analgesia/NSAIDs, steroid injection, physiotherapy, surgery.
Osteoarthritis	Inflammation of the shoulder joint.	Gradual onset of pain, stiffness and decreased movement of shoulder joint.	Tenderness on palpation of shoulder joint. Muscle weakness. Crepitus. Decreased ROM.	Due to wear and tear of the shoulder joint.	Analgesia/NSAIDs, steroid injection, physiotherapy, surgery.

Further management

- Refer urgently if suspected fracture, dislocation, nerve damage or red flags.
- Safety net – return to GP if not improving.
- Routine referral to orthopaedics for consideration of surgery/arthroscopy if non-surgical measures unsuccessful.

Role play

Information for doctor	Additional information for role player
Patient: Mr DF *Age*: 39 years *SH*: Lives alone. Unemployed. Smokes 20 cigs/day. Drinks 40 units alcohol/week. *FH*: Nil *PMH*: Nil *Information*: You are a salaried GP.	*PC*: *"I've done something to my shoulder".* *HPC*: Fell on left shoulder 6 weeks ago. Normally plays football weekly. Did improve but now has decreased movement of left shoulder. **Very painful around shoulder joint**. Pain mainly on movement. No swelling or numbness. **No night pain.** *ICE*: Would like to know the cause and would like painkillers. *O/E*: Tender on palpation around shoulder joint. Decreased abduction and internal rotation of shoulder. No swelling.

Knee pain

- Common causes of knee pain include meniscal, ligamentous or joint problems (osteoarthritis/rheumatoid arthritis/gout).
- Other common problems include patellar tendonitis, chondromalacia patellae, baker's cyst and Osgood–Schlatter disease.

Data gathering

Open question
- *"Can you describe in more detail the knee pain you've been experiencing?"*

Focused/closed questions

HPC: *"Where exactly are you experiencing the pain?"* *"Does the pain spread anywhere else?"*
"When did the pain first start?"
"Is it getting worse?"
"Is the pain worse at any particular time of the day?"
"Is there anything which makes the pain better or worse?"
"Did you injure your knee?"
"Have you ever injured your knee in the past?"
"Does your knee ever lock or give way?"
"Is there any swelling of your knee?"
"Are you still able to walk or run?"
"Do you have a fever?" (red flag)

PMH: Any previous knee problems or surgery?

FH: Any FH of joint problems?

SH: Who lives with you at home? Stairs at home? Occupation?

DH: *"Have you tried any painkillers for the pain so far?"*

ICE: *"Is there anything in particular you were hoping we could do to help?"*
"How does this pain affect you at home or at work?"

Examination: • Knee examination (see *Appendix 1*).

Clinical management

Investigations

- Blood tests – FBC, ESR, CRP, calcium, RhF.
- Fluid from knee aspirate for microscopy.
- Knee X-ray, USS or MRI.
- Knee arthroscopy – can diagnose joint problems and repair ligament or meniscal damage.

Explanation to patient and management

Common causes of knee pain	Description	History	Examination	Explanation to patient	Management
Osteoarthritis	Inflammation of the joints.	Gradual onset of pain, stiffness and limitation of joint movement.	Possible deformity and swelling of knee, decreased ROM, crepitus, decreased function.	Caused by wear and tear of the knee joint.	See Osteoarthritis section.
Meniscal problem	Damage to the menisci which help to lubricate and stabilise the knee joint.	Knee locking/ giving way. Medial or lateral knee pain. Often due to twisting injury.	Knee swelling +/- effusion. Decreased extension of knee. Pain or 'clicking' on twisting the knee during extension.	Menisci act like shock absorbers in the knee; can be torn commonly by a forceful twisting injury.	Analgesia +/- NSAIDs. Small tears may heal themselves. Larger tears require surgery.
Ligamentous injury	There are four ligaments which provide stability to the knee. These can be stretched, torn or ruptured usually by a forceful injury.	Pain, swelling and instability of the knee. Popping or snapping sound at the time of injury.	Swelling and tenderness around the knee joint. Effusion in knee. Decreased ROM. Anterior/ posterior draw test and Lachman test may be +ve.	Ligaments are strong tissues around joints which connect bone together. Ligaments can be injured usually by being stretched during a sudden pull.	Analgesia/ NSAIDs. Rest, immobilisation, physiotherapy, surgery.

Common causes of knee pain	Description	History	Examination	Explanation to patient	Management
Patellar tendonitis	Inflammation of the patellar tendon where it attaches to the patella. Can progress to tearing and degeneration of the tendon.	Pain over the patella usually due to overuse injury from repetitive overloading, e.g. jumping.	Knee swelling. Patellar tenderness on palpation. Pain on extension/ flexion of the knee.	Inflammation of the fibrous tissue that connects muscle to bone around the knee cap.	Rest, activity modification, NSAIDs, strengthening exercises, steroid joint injection.
Chondro-malacia patellae	Softening of articular cartilage of the patella.	Common in young girls. Usually due to indirect trauma. Usually anterior knee pain worse on rising and using stairs.	Patellar tenderness, crepitus, fluid behind the knee. Pain on passive movements of the knee.	Irritation of the undersurface of the knee cap.	Avoid repetitive knee bending and excessive activity. Immobilisation, analgesia/ NSAIDs, knee supports, surgery.
Osgood–Schlatter's	Inflammation of the tibial tubercle due to overuse and excessive force acting on this bone.	Occurs in teenagers, especially boys. Pain and swelling just below the knee, worse after activity and eases with rest.	Tender bony lump and swelling below the knee cap. Normal ROM.	Bony protrusion below the knee becomes inflamed.	Ease off strenuous sport, ice pack, knee support, simple analgesia, physiotherapy.
Baker's cyst	Benign swelling of the semi-membranous bursa behind the knee joint.	Pain and swelling at the back of the knee. Knee locking.	Transilluminable swelling in the popliteal space.	Fluid-filled swelling that develops at the back of the knee.	May self resolve with no treatment or NSAIDs. RICE. Occasionally steroid injection or surgery.

Role play

Information for doctor	Additional information for role player
Patient: Mrs SK *Age*: 58 years *SH*: Lives with husband. Has stairs at home. Receptionist. *FH*: Diabetes *PMH*: Diabetes *DH*: Metformin 500 mg BD, gliclazide 40 mg OD *Information*: You are a locum GP.	*PC*: *"I've got terrible pain in my right knee".* *HPC*: Right knee pain for the past few weeks. No trauma. Pain over patella and medial side. **Worse after walking. Knee sometimes gives way. No locking.** No swelling of knee. **Has tried paracetamol and ibuprofen so far but still painful**. *ICE*: Would like a scan and would like some stronger painkillers. *O/E*: No swelling or effusion. Tenderness around medial joint line. Some crepitus on flexion of knee. Normal ROM. Decreased extension of right knee.

Osteoarthritis

- Inflammation of the joints resulting in pain and stiffness.
- Commonly affects hips, knees and hands.
- Treatment includes analgesia, physiotherapy or surgery (joint replacement).

Data gathering

Open question

- *"Can you tell me more about the pain you've been experiencing?"*

Focused/closed questions

HPC: *"Where exactly is the pain?" "Does the pain spread anywhere else?"*
"When did it start?" "Is it getting worse?"
"Is the pain worse at any particular time of the day?"
"Were there any triggers for the pain?"
"Are any other joints affected?"
"Does anything make the pain better/worse?"
"Any fever or weight loss?" (red flags)
"Is the pain affecting your sleep?"

PMH: Any previous injuries or joint problems?

FH: Any FH of arthritis?

SH: Smoking/alcohol history? Occupation? Who lives with you at home?

ICE: *"What do you think is causing this pain?"*
"How is it impacting on your quality of life?"

Examination:
- Joint examination (see *Appendix 1*).
- Function and gait assessment.

Clinical management

Investigations

- X-ray.
- Blood test – FBC, ESR, rheumatology screen, urate (to rule out other causes for joint pain).

Explanation to patient

- A joint is where two bones meet, and there is a hard smooth tissue called cartilage which covers the ends of the bones at the joint. There is also a fluid surrounding the joint called synovial fluid that helps to lubricate the joint.
- In osteoarthritis, the joint cartilage becomes damaged and worn, and the bone around the cartilage can also be damaged.

Management

(based on *NICE*, 2014, *CG177: Osteoarthritis*)

- Conservative management – weight loss, exercise and local muscle strengthening, walking aids, sensible footwear, splints/braces.
- Other non-pharmacological treatment – consider the use of TENS, do not offer glucosamine and chondroitin, do not offer acupuncture.
- Pharmacological management – paracetamol and topical NSAIDs first line. If insufficient, then consider addition of opioids or NSAIDs.
- Other treatments include intra-articular steroid injections, physiotherapy +/– occupational therapy.
- Safety net – return if symptoms not improving.
- Refer for surgery if non-surgical treatments have failed.

Role play

Information for doctor		Additional information for role player
Patient:	Mrs PS	*PC*: "*I have come to discuss my hip X-ray results*".
Age:	73 years	*HPC*: Left hip pain which is mainly worse at the end
SH:	Lives in a residential home.	of the day after walking. **No radiation down**
PMH:	Blindness, hypertension.	**the leg. Affects ability to walk.** No trauma. No
DH:	Bendrofluazide 2.5 mg OD.	other joints affected. **No weight loss or fever.**
Information:	Last consultation 2 weeks ago – left hip	**Has tried paracetamol and a heat pad so far –**
	pain for several months. X-ray left hip –	**no improvement.**
	joint space narrowing, osteophytes.	*FH*: Nil.
		ICE: Hoping for some painkillers and wants to know
		diagnosis.

Osteoporosis

- Occurs when a person's bones are less dense than normal and more prone to fractures.
- About 1 in 3 women over the age of 50 are thought to have osteoporosis.
- Osteoporosis results in about 60 000 hip fractures a year in the UK (*Ann R Coll Surg Engl*, 2008; 90: 213)
- Risk factors for osteoporosis include early menopause, family history, low body mass index, smokers, alcohol excess, patients on long-term steroids and those who have a sedentary lifestyle.
- Fracture risk assessment should therefore be considered in patients with any of the above risk factors or in women >65 years, men >75 years. This can be done using FRAX or Q Fracture. Once 10-year absolute fracture risk is calculated, those at high risk should be offered treatment and lifestyle advice. Those at intermediate risk should be referred for DEXA scan.
- Management includes bisphosphonates and lifestyle measures.

Data gathering

Open questions
- *"What problems have you been experiencing with your bones?"*
- *"What do you understand about your recent DEXA scan results?"*

Focused/closed questions
HPC: *"Have you ever fractured any bones before?"*
"Do you have any bone pains?"
"Have you had any recent falls?"
"At what age did you go through the menopause?"
"Have you noticed any weight loss or night sweats?" (red flags)

PMH: *"Do you have any history of bone problems?"* *"Do you have any illnesses such as diabetes or inflammatory bowel disease?"*

FH: *"Is there a history of osteoporosis or hip fractures in your family?"* *"Is there a family history of early menopause?"*

DH: Are you on any regular medications? Have you ever been on long term steroids?

SH: Smoking/alcohol history? Diet/exercise?

ICE: *"What concerns do you have about your bones?"*

Examination: • BMI.
• Examine bone/joint if pain.

Clinical management

Investigations
- Calculate FRAX or Q Fracture risk.
- DEXA scan if intermediate risk.

- Blood test – FBC, U&Es, TFTs, calcium, phosphate, vitamin D, LFTs, ALP, LH, FSH, testosterone.

Explanation to patient

- A DEXA scan uses X-rays to determine how strong your bones are.
- DEXA scan result varies from normal bone strength, osteopenia (slightly weaker bones than normal) and osteoporosis.
- If a DEXA scan shows you have osteoporosis, you may be given advice and treatment to try strengthening your bones.
- Bisphosphonates are commonly used and these help to slow the rate of bone loss.

Management

- Conservative management – increase dietary calcium intake, reduce alcohol and increase weight bearing exercise.
- Stop smoking.
- Consider reducing or stopping steroids if on steroid therapy.
- Calcium and vitamin D (for all at risk of falls or in residential care)
- HRT should be offered if premature menopause to reduce risk of osteoporotic fracture.

NICE recommendations for primary and secondary prevention of osteoporosis
(2008, *TA160/161: Osteoporosis*)

- Alendronate is recommended as first line if the patient fulfils the criteria for treatment (post-menopausal women with previous fragility fracture, >70 years on high dose steroids, post-menopausal women and men >50 years at high risk of osteoporotic fracture). This can be continued for 10 years.
- Risedronate can be used when alendronate cannot be tolerated. Zoledronate and denosumab can be used for those intolerant of standard oral bisphosphonates (which can cause oesophagitis, AF and osteonecrosis of the jaw).
- Strontium is contraindicated in those with CV disease.
- Consider a repeat DEXA after 3 years to assess response to treatment.

Role play

Information for doctor	Additional information for role player
Patient: Mrs ER *Age*: 64 years *PMH*: Breast cancer 2008 *DH*: Nil *Information*: Had a DEXA scan 2 weeks ago. Results – spinal T score 1.1; hip T score – 2.8.	*PC*: "*I have come for the results of my bone scan I had recently*". *HPC*: Had a Colles fracture 2 months ago following a fall. No bone pain at present. Reached menopause aged 54 years. **Previous ankle fracture 2 years ago.** *FH*: **Mum and sister had osteoporosis.** *ICE*: Thinks she may have osteoporosis so keen to start taking medication to protect the bones as this is what her sister took. *O/E*: BMI 19

Rheumatoid arthritis

- Common form of arthritis resulting in pain, swelling and inflammation of the joints.
- Most commonly develops between the ages of 40 and 60 years.
- Rheumatoid arthritis (RA) is an independent risk factor for CVD, increasing risk of CV mortality by up to 50%.
- It is thought to be caused by an autoimmune process.
- Typically causes symmetrical joint synovitis of small joints of hands and feet.
- NICE guidelines 2015 encourage early referral if RA suspected – urgently (within 2 weeks) if small joints of hands or feet involved, >1 joint involved or >3 months since onset of symptoms.
- Treatment includes disease-modifying drugs to suppress inflammation, analgesia and surgery in severe cases.
- The figure below shows a simple diagram that you can use to illustrate rheumatoid arthritis to your patients.

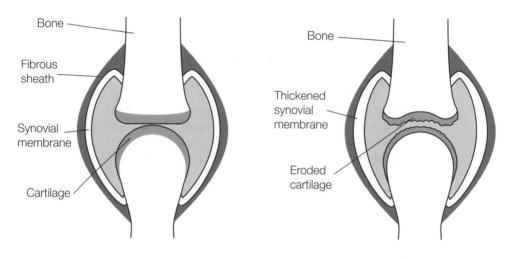

Data gathering

Open question

- *"Can you tell me more about your joint problems?"*

Focused/closed questions

HPC: *"Which joints are affected?"*
"Are both sides affected?"
"When did the problems first start?" "Have the problems been getting worse?"
"Do you have any pain or swelling in the joints?"
"Any injury to your joints?"
"Is it worse at any particular time of the day?"

"Have you noticed any fever or weight loss or muscle pains?" (red flags)
"Have you had any eye or chest symptoms?"

FH: Any FH of rheumatoid arthritis?

DH: Are you currently taking any medication?

SH: Occupation? Who lives with you at home? *"Are you managing OK at home?"*

ICE: *"What concerns do you have about the joint pains?"*
"Does it stop you from doing the things you would normally be able to do?"

Examination: • Joint examination.

Clinical management

Investigations

- Blood test – rheumatoid factor* (present in two-thirds of people with RA), CRP, FBC (*can also be used to monitor disease control).
- X-ray (particularly if hands and feet affected).
- If RA strongly suspected do not delay referral whilst awaiting blood results or if results are normal.

Explanation to patient

- Arthritis means inflammation of the joints where two bones meet.
- In rheumatoid arthritis, the immune system makes antibodies against the tissues that surround each joint. This causes inflammation around the affected joint, and the cartilage which lines the joint can become eroded. Over time, this joint damage causes deformities of the joints.
- The main symptoms are pain and stiffness of the affected joints, and this is usually worse in the morning.

Management

- Patients should be referred to secondary care urgently if RA suspected. DMARDs will usually be commenced early if diagnosis confirmed. Steroids are also often used and are particularly helpful in managing a flare of RA, but should NOT be prescribed in primary care before diagnosis confirmed at specialist review.
- MDT approach is encouraged with patients given access to a named member such as a specialist nurse.
- NSAIDs and analgesia.
- Steroids, e.g. prednisolone, for flare-ups.
- Physical activity.
- Physiotherapy +/– occupational therapy. This should include 'hand exercise programmes', if appropriate, once disease is stable.
- Assess CV risk of all patients with QRISK2–2015 and consider statin therapy.
- Osteoporosis risk is also increased therefore check FRAX or Q Fracture and consider bone protection.
- Once diagnosed, ensure patient has named access to MDT. They should return to GP if symptoms not improving. Patient also requires drug monitoring if on methotrexate.
- Surgery can be offered for deformity, pain and loss of function if other treatments unsuccessful.

Role play

Information for doctor	Additional information for role player
Patient: Mrs AF	*PC*: *"I've been getting a lot of pain in my hands, and I'm struggling a bit".*
Age: 70 years	
SH: Lives alone in 1 bed house with no carers.	*HPC*: Worsening pain for the past few months in both hands. Also stiffness worse in the morning. Right thumb and index fingers are the worst affected. No trauma. No muscle pains, fever or eye symptoms.
FH: Mother and grandmother had RA	
PMH: TIA 2007; hypercholesterolaemia	
DH: Simvastatin 40 mg OD, aspirin 75 mg OD	
	ICE: **Difficulty at home especially with cooking and cleaning. Would like some extra help.**
Information: Recently saw practice nurse for influenza vaccination. You are a GP Registrar.	*O/E*: Swelling and deformity of both hands, especially right hand. No erythema or hot joints. Unable to fasten buttons or open jar lid with right hand.

Polymyalgia rheumatica

- Condition caused by inflammation of the large muscles.
- Causes pain and stiffness mainly in the muscles of the neck, shoulders and hips.
- It mainly affects people over the age of 65 and low dose steroids help to ease the symptoms.

Data gathering

Open question

- *"Tell me a bit more about the muscle pain and stiffness you have been getting."*

Focused/closed questions

HPC: *"Do you have any muscle pain or stiffness?" "If so, which muscles are affected?" "Is the pain on both sides?" "Is the pain and/or stiffness worse at any particular time of the day?"* (usually worse first thing in the morning with PMR)

"How long have you had these symptoms for?"

"Have you had any difficulty getting up from bed or from a chair?"

"Have you had any difficulty combing your hair?"

"Have you had any swelling of your hands, feet or joints?"

"Do you have any visual loss and/or headache?" (red flag – possible temporal arteritis)

"Have you had any pain in your jaw when chewing?" (red flag)

"Have you had any tiredness, loss of appetite or weight loss?"

DH: *"Do you take any regular medications?"* (avoid NSAIDs with steroids)

SH: *"Who lives with you at home?" "Do you have adequate help at home?"* Occupation?

ICE: *"How are you coping with work/daily life?"*

Examination:
- Examination of neck, shoulders and/or hips.
- Palpation of temporal arteries.

Clinical management

Investigations
- Blood test – ESR, CRP. Also perform FBC, U&E, LFT, calcium, CK and TSH to exclude other causes.
- If suspecting temporal arteritis, refer urgently for possible temporal artery biopsy.

Explanation to patient
- Polymyalgia rheumatica (PMR) is a condition causing inflammation of the large muscles in the body.
- There is commonly pain and stiffness in the muscles around the shoulder, neck, upper arms and hips.
- The symptoms typically develop gradually over a few days or weeks.
- A steroid medicine called prednisolone is usually given to reduce the inflammation and ease the symptoms, and this medication will usually be needed for 2–3 years.
- Approximately 30% of people with PMR also develop a condition called temporal arteritis, resulting in inflammation of the arteries that pass over the temples. If this isn't treated promptly it can result in blindness.

Management
- Prednisolone – start with 15 mg daily and reduce slowly to a maintenance dose of about 5 mg daily.
- If features of GCA develop, increase prednisolone to 40–60 mg and refer urgently.
- Refer if atypical features or doubts about diagnosis – consider referral for methotrexate if steroids needed for >2 years.
- Ensure patient carries a steroid card if on regular steroids.
- Osteoporosis prophylaxis if at increased risk.

Role play

Information for doctor	Additional information for role player
Patient: Mrs AW *Age*: 70 years *SH*: Retired. Widowed. **Lives with son.** *PMH*: Osteoporosis *DH*: Alendronic acid 70 mg once weekly, calcichew D3 forte 1 tab BD *Information*: You are a salaried GP.	*PC*: *"I've been feeling very achey and stiff for the past couple of weeks"* *HPC*: Having difficulty getting up from her chair. Pain mainly around shoulders and hips, and worse in morning. **No visual loss, headache or pain when chewing. Tiredness but no weight loss.** *ICE*: Son helps but is at work during the day and she struggles when on her own. *O/E*: Pain and stiffness on active and passive movements of the shoulder and hip – worse on resisted movement. Temporal arteries not palpable and no tenderness around temples.

Tennis elbow

- This was previously also known as lateral epicondylitis but is now termed extensor tendinopathy.
- Most commonly seen in the 30–50 year age group.
- Causes pain on the lateral side of the elbow, which often improves with rest, pain relief and/or physiotherapy.

Data gathering

Open question

- *"Can you tell me more about the elbow pain you have been experiencing?"*

Focused/closed questions

HPC: *"Where exactly are you experiencing the pain?" "Does the pain radiate?"*
"Is the pain on both sides?"
"When did the pain start?"
"Is the pain present all the time or does it come and go?"
"Do you know what might have triggered the pain?"
"Did you injure your elbow?"
"Have you tried any treatments so far?"
"Any swelling of the elbow?"
"Any fever?" (red flag)

SH: Occupation? Smoking/alcohol/illicit drug history? *"Do you play any sports regularly?" "Is there anyone at home who can help you if you need assistance?"*

ICE: *"What were you hoping we might be able to do to help?"*
"Has the pain stopped you from doing anything that you would usually do?"

Examination: • Elbow examination (see *Appendix 1*).

Clinical management

Investigations

- Initially clinical diagnosis.
- If not improving consider MRI scan.

Explanation to patient

- Tennis elbow occurs due to inflammation of the tissue (the tendons) that connects the muscle to the bone at the elbow.
- It causes pain in the outer part of the elbow, and it is often worse with twisting movements of the arm (e.g. opening a jar).

- The pain is often caused by an injury to one or more of the tendons around the elbow. The injuries are often caused by overuse of the forearm, particularly seen in manual workers and racquet sports players.

Management

- Rest or modify activities that bring on the symptoms – normally self limiting condition.
- Analgesia (e.g. paracetamol, NSAIDs, codeine phosphate), GTN patches.
- Steroid injection (Botox injections may also have a role).
- Physiotherapy – eccentric exercises of the wrist extensor tendon help to elongate the tendon.
- Elbow support or splint.
- Safety net – return to GP if above measures not helping.
- Referral for surgery (to remove the damaged part of the tendon) if non-surgical treatments unsuccessful.

Role play

Information for doctor		Additional information for role player	
Patient:	Mr PS	*PC*:	*"I have been having trouble with my right elbow".*
Age:	37 years	*HPC*:	Pain in the right elbow for the past month.
SH:	Married with one child. Joiner. Non-smoker, 5 units alcohol/week.		Pain mainly on the lateral side. No radiation. Intermittent pain. **Worse when working**.
FH:	Nil		Has tried paracetamol and diclofenac but no
PMH:	Arthroscopy of left knee 2008		improvement. Slight swelling of the elbow.
Information:	You are a salaried GP.		**Plays squash once a week but now difficult due to pain.**
		ICE:	**Would like to know what is causing it, and would like some stronger painkillers.**
		O/E:	Afebrile. Tenderness over right lateral epicondyle. Pain worse on supination of the right arm.

Carpal tunnel syndrome

- Pain and/or numbness of the hand, as a result of compression of the median nerve as it passes through the carpal tunnel at the wrist.
- A ligament called the retinaculum lies across the front of the wrist, and the carpal tunnel is the space between this ligament and the bones of the wrist.
- The figure below shows a simple diagram that you can use to illustrate carpal tunnel syndrome to your patients.
- Management includes analgesia, wrist splint, steroid injection or surgery.

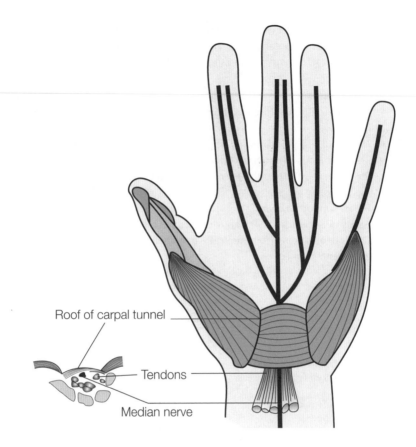

Roof of carpal tunnel

Tendons

Median nerve

Data gathering

Open question

- *"Can you tell me about the problem with your hand?"*

Focused/closed questions

HPC: *"When did the problem first start?"*

"Do you have any pain, numbness, burning, tingling or weakness in your hand?"

"Which fingers are specifically affected?"

"Are the symptoms worse at any particular time of the day?"

"Are you aware of any aggravating or relieving factors?"

"Have you noticed any wasting of your hand muscles?" (red flag)

"Did you injure your hand?"

"Do the symptoms wake you up at night?"

"Have you noticed your hand is weak?"

PMH: Any history of arthritis or wrist problems? Any history of thyroid problems or diabetes? Are you pregnant?

FH: Any family history of carpal tunnel syndrome?

SH: Occupation? Manual work? Smoking/alcohol/illicit drug history?

ICE: *"What do you think is causing your symptoms?"*

Examination:
- Weight.
- Examination of the hand – check for muscle wasting, tenderness, thumb abduction, power and sensation.
- Phalen's test – press the back of the hands together, flexing the wrists. The test is positive if the patient experiences tingling or increased numbness within 1 minute.
- Tinel's test – tap or press on the median nerve at the wrist. The test is positive if you experience tingling or a shock-like sensation.

Clinical management

Investigation
- FBC, U&Es, TFTs, CRP, ESR, fasting glucose (to check for possible causes).
- Nerve conduction studies or EMG may be considered if the diagnosis is uncertain or if surgery is being considered.

Explanation to patient
- Carpal tunnel syndrome is caused by pressure on a nerve around the wrist.
- The nerve involved is the median nerve which supplies sensation to the thumb, index and middle fingers, and half of the ring finger. It also controls some of the movements of the thumb.

Management
- Leave alone – often resolves without any treatment. Return to GP if no improvement.
- Conservative management – weight loss, avoid over-use of the wrist, wrist splint.
- There is no evidence that NSAIDs or diuretics are effective..
- Steroid injection – reduces inflammation.
- Surgery – the ligament is cut to ease the pressure on the carpal tunnel.
- If thenar muscle wasting the patient must be referred to orthopaedics.

Role play

Information for doctor	Additional information for role player
Patient: Mrs RJ *Age*: 78 years *SH*: Lives alone, widowed, retired *PMH*: Rheumatoid arthritis *DH*: Naproxen 250 mg BD *Information*: Last consultation 1 month ago due to arthritic pain. You are a GP partner.	*PC*: Tingling in left hand and painful left wrist. *HPC*: Two month history but symptoms worsening. **No trauma.** Numbness of left thumb, index and middle finger. Worse at the end of the day. **Left handed. Weakness of left hand also. Shaking helps to relieve tingling.** *ICE*: Worried about cause of tingling. **Restricts day to day tasks – pain when opening jars, etc.** *O/E*: Reduced sensation in lateral three digits. Tinel's test positive. No thenar muscle wasting.

Dermatology

Eczema

- Atopic eczema describes a chronic inflammatory itchy skin condition which usually develops in early childhood.
- Typically the skin becomes dry and inflamed.
- The cause is not fully known, although it is thought that the oily barrier of the skin is reduced, making the skin more susceptible to irritants and allergens.
- Approximately 2 in 3 children with atopic eczema grow out of it by mid teens.
- The most commonly affected areas are the skin creases and around the neck. The face is commonly affected in babies.
- Treatments include emollients and topical steroids for flare-ups.

Data gathering

Open question
- *"What problems have you been experiencing with your skin?"*

Focused/closed questions

HPC: *"When did you first develop problems with your skin?"*
"How often do you get flare-ups?"
"Does your skin get dry and/or itchy?"
"Which areas of your skin are affected?"
"Do you have any infected and/or weepy areas?"
"Does it affect your sleep?"
"Have you noticed any blistering of your skin?" (red flag)
"Do you have any painful areas of skin?" (red flag)
"Have you had any fever?" (red flag)
"Have you had any joint pains?"
"Are you aware of any particular triggers, for example, certain foods?"
"Any concerns with growth and development?" (child)

FH: Any FH of eczema, hayfever or asthma?

SH: *"What is your job?"* *"Any exposure to chemicals or other skin irritants in the workplace?"*

DH: *"What treatments have you already tried for your skin?"*

ICE: *"What were you hoping we could do to help with your skin?"*
"How has it been affecting you?"

Examination: • Skin examination – distribution (symmetrical/asymmetrical, flexors/extensors), erythema, scaling, crusting, weeping, excoriation, vesicles, pustules, scarring.

Clinical management

Investigations
- No specific investigations.
- If possible unknown allergic trigger consider skin prick testing.

Explanation to patient
- Eczema is inflammation of the skin which is often dry and itchy and it can flare up from time to time.
- Sometimes the inflamed areas can become weepy and infected.
- The cause is not fully known although it does run in families and it is also thought to be caused by a problem with the immune system.

Management
- Patient education including written information.
- Avoid allergens, e.g. perfumes or detergents including soaps and bubble baths as they can be skin irritants.
- Avoid scratching and wear cotton clothing.
- Antihistamines or crotamiton cream to reduce the itching (not routinely recommended, however).
- Use non-biological detergents.
- NICE advises a trial of hypoallergenic formula in infants with moderate to severe eczema in whom cow's milk protein allergy is suspected.
- Emollients (use liberally at least 2–4 times daily) and soap substitutes.
- Topical corticosteroids for short term use for flare-ups (e.g. 1% hydrocortisone).
- The evidence supports the use of tacrolimus for short-term, intermittent treatment of moderate to severe atopic eczema that has not been controlled by topical corticosteroids.
- Antibiotics either topically or orally for infected eczema (e.g. fusidic acid cream or oral flucloxacillin).
- Safety net – return if not improving.
- If suspected eczema herpeticum refer immediately to hospital (areas of rapidly worsening, painful eczema, with blisters or ulcerated lesions and possible fever).
- Routine dermatology referral if uncertain diagnosis, poor response to treatment, or if associated with severe or recurrent infections (*NICE*, 2007, *CG57: Atopic eczema in children*).

Role play

Information for doctor	Additional information for role player
Patient: Ms SM *Age*: 17 years *SH*: College student, lives with parents *PMH*: Eczema *DH*: Cetraben emollient cream BD, hydrocortisone 1% cream PRN *Information*: You are a locum GP.	*PC*: Flare-up of eczema in the last few days, which isn't settling with emollients and hydrocortisone. Dry, itchy skin on back of knees, hands and arms. **No weeping or blistering. No fever. No known trigger.** *FH*: **Sister and mum have eczema and asthma.** *ICE*: Would like some other cream to control the eczema. *O/E*: Scaly, red, inflamed patches especially on popliteal fossa and hands. Some excoriation and weeping areas on the forearms.

Psoriasis

- Skin condition that typically results in plaques of red, scaly skin.
- There are different types of psoriasis, but plaque psoriasis is the commonest type.
- Other types include scalp, nail, guttate, flexural, pustular or erythrodermic psoriasis.
- There is no cure, but treatments include emollients, vitamin D based creams, coal tar preparations, dithranol and steroid creams.

Data gathering

Open question
- *"Can you tell me more about the skin problems you are having?"*

Focused/closed questions
HPC: *"Where specifically have you got the skin problem?"*
"When did it develop?" "How has it progressed?"
"Have you tried any treatments so far?"
"Were there any triggers?"
"Is your skin itchy?" "Is your skin painful or sore?"
"Have you noticed any nail or scalp changes?"
"Any pain in your joints?" (red flag)
"Have you noticed lots of fluid-filled spots on your skin?" (red flag – widespread pustular psoriasis)

PMH: Any previous skin problems? Any medical conditions? Any recent illness/infections?

FH: Any family history of psoriasis?

SH: Smoking/alcohol/illicit drug history? Occupation? Stress?

DH: *"Are you on any medications?"* (beta blockers, NSAIDs and ACE inhibitors can trigger or worsen psoriasis)

ICE: *"What do you think is causing this skin rash?"*

Examination:
- Inspection of skin, scalp and nails:
  - skin – distribution, erythema, macules, papules, plaques, pustules (commonest presentation is well defined scaly erythematous plaques on extensor surfaces)
  - scalp – erythematous plaques, scales
  - nails – pitting, yellow discolouration, onycholysis.
- Joint examination.
- Eye examination – inspection of lids, conjunctiva and cornea.

Clinical management

Investigations
- No specific investigations recommended.
- Occasionally a skin biopsy is done.
- Use the dermatology Quality of Life Index score to assess the impact. A score of ≥5 should prompt a referral.
- Assess for psoriatic arthritis using the Psoriasis Epidemiology Screening (PEST) Tool.

Explanation to patient
- Psoriasis is a skin condition that occurs because there is a faster turnover of skin cells than usual. This results in a build up of cells on the top layer of skin, which causes plaques to form. It is not clearly understood why this occurs. There is also some skin inflammation that occurs.
- Aggravating factors include stress, infections, drugs, smoking, sunlight and injury to the skin.
- Some people with psoriasis will also get joint and nail problems.
- Psoriasis can flare up from time to time and there is no definite cure.

Management
(based on *NICE, 2012, CG153: Psoriasis*)
- Conservative treatments – avoid stressors, stop smoking, healthy diet, exercise, support groups.
- Emollients – softens hardened plaques.
- First line treatments:
  - Vitamin D based creams (calcipitriol, calcitriol) – reduce the rate of cell division of the skin cells.
  - Steroid creams – reduce inflammation.
- Second line treatment: coal tar, which reduces turnover of the skin cells and reduces inflammation. Can be used for plaque psoriasis or for scalp psoriasis in combination with salicylic acid preparations.
- Dithranol (a specialist option for treatment-resistant psoriasis)– reduces plaque formation.
- Nail psoriasis – topical corticosteroids +/– salicylic acid or vitamin D analogue.

- If poor response to the above treatments refer to dermatologist for consideration of PUVA (ultraviolet light treatment) or other specialist treatments.
- Safety net – patients with suspected widespread pustular psoriasis (erythroderma) should be referred to hospital immediately because it is potentially fatal.

Role play

Information for doctor	Additional information for role player
Patient: Mr JS *Age*: 40 years *SH*: Married with 2 children. Builder. Smokes 20 cigs/day. *PMH*: Nil *DH*: Nil *Information*: No previous consultations. You are a locum GP.	*PC*: *"I have had a problem with my skin for the past month".* *HPC*: Dry itchy skin, mainly on the elbows. Improved when I went on holiday to Spain last week but still present. **No painful joints. No scalp or nail changes. Tried E45 cream but no improvement.** *FH*: Father has psoriasis. *ICE*: Thinks it may also be psoriasis. Would like some cream to get rid of it as looks unsightly. *O/E*: Erythematous scaly plaques on both elbows.

Acne

- Common cause of skin problems, especially amongst teenagers.
- Causes spots to develop, usually affecting the face, but can also affect the back, neck and chest.
- The spots can range from blackheads and whiteheads which are often mild, to inflamed pus-filled pustules and cysts, which can be severe and long lasting and can lead to scarring.
- Treatment includes topical preparations, retinoids, antibiotics or the combined oral contraceptive pill.

Data gathering

Open question
- *"Can you describe the problems that you have been having with your skin?"*

Focused/closed questions
HPC: *"How long have you had the spots for?"* *"Are they getting worse?"*
"Have you noticed any triggers for the spots?"
"Have you tried any over-the-counter treatments?"
"Where do you get the spots?"
"Do you have spots on other parts of your body?"
"Have you noticed any weight gain, facial hair or changes to your periods?" (possible PCOS in females)

FH: *"Does anyone else in the family have acne or any other skin problems?"*

SH: Smoking/alcohol/illicit drug history? Occupation? *"How does this affect your social life and relationships?"*

DH: Are you taking any other medications? (progesterone only contraceptives, steroids, lithium and anti-convulsants can worsen acne)

ICE: *"How does your skin problem affect you?" "How does it affect your self esteem?"*

Examination: • Skin examination – inspection for erythema, hyperpigmentation, papules, pustules, comedones and scarring.

Clinical management

Investigations
- Nothing specific.

Explanation to patient
- Acne is caused by a problem with the glands beneath the skin that make sebum (oil).
- Some pores become blocked and the sebum becomes trapped. This can result in bacteria multiplying in these blocked pores. Inflammation can then occur in the surrounding skin.

Management
- Conservative management – avoid any possible triggers or aggravating factors, e.g. cosmetic products or certain drugs. Avoid picking or squeezing spots.
- Topical preparations, e.g. benzoyl peroxide, retinoids (e.g. adapalene*), azelaic acid, antibiotics.
- Antibiotic tablets, e.g. tetracycline, lymecycline (minimum 3–6 month course). Never use with topical antibiotics to reduce resistance.
- Combined oral contraceptive pill, e.g. Dianette.
- Referral to specialist if poor response to treatment or in severe cases of acne.

*mainstay of treatment now instead of antibiotics due to the development of resistance.

Role play

Information for doctor		Additional information for role player
Patient:	Mr TW	*PC*: Acne.
Age:	16 years	*HPC*: Acne not improving with medication given. No known triggers. Has spots on face and back.
PMH:	Nil	
DH:	Benzoyl peroxide BD	*SH*: Lives with parents and younger sister.
FH:	Nil	*ICE*: **Feels self-conscious about his skin. Starting college soon and keen to get problem sorted.**
Information:	Last consultation with GP 3 months ago – problem with acne. You are a salaried GP.	*O/E*: Moderate pustular and nodular acne on the face and back.

Endocrinology

Diabetes

- Diabetes mellitus is a long-term condition which occurs when the level of glucose in the blood becomes higher than normal.
- There are two main types of diabetes mellitus – type 1 and type 2.
- In type 1 diabetes the beta cells in the pancreas stop producing insulin, and the blood glucose level increases.
- In type 2 diabetes you still make insulin, but either you do not make enough for your body's needs or the cells in your body are unable to use this insulin properly.
- The NICE 2015 guidelines for type 2 diabetes recommend adopting an individualized approach to diabetes care, taking into account factors such as patient preference, co-morbidities, polypharmacy and life expectancy.

Data gathering

Open question
- *"Can you tell me more about your symptoms and when it all started?"*

Focused/closed questions

HPC: *"Have you got any increased thirst or are you passing urine more than usual?"*
"Have you had any weight loss?"
"How have your energy levels been?"
"Have these symptoms been getting worse?"
"Have you suffered with recurrent thrush or other infections?"
"Have you noticed any problems with your vision?"
"Do you have any problems with the sensation in your feet?"
"Any problems with chest pain or any shortness of breath?" (red flags)
"Any vomiting, problems breathing or confusion?" (red flags – DKA/HONK)

FH: Any family history of diabetes?

PMH: Do you have any other medical conditions, e.g. hypothyroidism?

DH: Do you take any regular medications? Diuretics?

SH: Smoking/alcohol/illicit drug history? Occupation? Do you drive? Diet/exercise?

ICE: *"What do you think is causing these symptoms?"*

Examination:
- BP, pulse, respiratory rate.
- BMI.
- Visual acuity/fundoscopy.
- Foot examination including peripheral pulses.

Clinical management

Investigations
- Urinalysis – check for glucose, ketones and microalbuminuria.
- Bloods – HbA1C, FBC, U&Es. If HbA1C >48, repeat in 2–4 weeks for confirmation if asymptomatic. If HbA1C 42–47 diagnose pre-diabetes, provide lifestyle advice and repeat in 1 year.

Explanation to patient
- Normally, the amount of sugar in the blood is controlled by a hormone called insulin, which is produced by the pancreas.
- When food is digested and enters the bloodstream, insulin moves any sugar out of the blood and into cells, where it is broken down to produce energy.
- In people with diabetes mellitus, the body is unable to break down sugar into energy because there is not enough insulin or the insulin doesn't work properly. If the sugar level remains poorly controlled, this can result in various problems including eye, feet, and kidney problems, and there is an increased risk of developing heart disease or stroke.

Management
(based on *NICE*, 2015, *NG28: Type 2 diabetes in adults*)
- Refer to A&E immediately if any signs of DKA or HONK (glycosuria or ketonuria with tachycardia, hypotension, dehydration or altered level of consciousness).
- Monitor HbA1C every 2–6 months until stable and then annually thereafter (aim for below 48 mmol/mol, although targets should be individualised, e.g. higher levels may be appropriate for frail patients to prevent hypoglycaemia).
- Healthy diet – high fibre, low glycaemic index sources of carbohydrate. Low fat dairy products and oily fish. Control intake of saturated fats.
- Exercise, weight control, smoking cessation.
- Self-monitor plasma glucose for those on insulin, oral hypoglycaemics or to monitor changes during intercurrent illness.
- BP control (aim for <140/80 mmHg or <130/80 mmHg if kidney, eye or cerebrovascular damage):
  - Lifestyle advice – low salt diet, exercise.
  - ACE inhibitor or ARB if <55 years, or of African or Caribbean descent at any age.
  - Monitor BP 6 monthly if stable, more frequently if not.
- Annual eye, foot and kidney function checks (or more frequently if any abnormalities detected).
- Lipid management:
  - Aim for total cholesterol <4.0 mmol/l and LDL <2.0 mmol/l.

- Offer atorvastatin 20 mg nocte for primary prevention if >10% 10-year CV risk using QRISK2-2015.
- Offer atorvastatin 80 mg nocte for secondary prevention.
- If target cholesterol still not reached, increase atorvastatin or try another statin or ezetimibe. Seek specialist advice if TG >10mmol/l, urgently if TG >20 mmol/l.
- Offer low dose aspirin only if established CV disease.
- Patient education programme and/or support group.

Type 1 diabetes
- Insulin.
- Referral to specialist diabetic nurse or endocrinologist at diagnosis.
- Aim for pre-prandial blood glucose level of 4–7 mmol/l and post-prandial level of <9 mmol/l.

Type 2 diabetes
- Diet, weight control and exercise.
- If HbA1C still 48 mmol/l or above, start metformin 500 mg OD and titrate as required (introduce slowly to minimize GI side effects; also monitor U&Es & LFTs).
- First intensification of treatment to dual therapy is suggested at 58 mmol/mol, aiming for a target of 53 mmol/mol. Drugs which can be considered include gliptins, pioglitazone, sulphonylureas or SGLT2 inhibitors.
- If HbA1C is still >58 mmol/mol on dual therapy, then NICE suggests a second intensification of treatment to triple therapy, again aiming for a target of 53 mmol/mol.
- If HbA1C ≥58 despite maximum tolerated oral medication, consider adding insulin.

Role play

Information for doctor	Additional information for role player
Patient: Mr JH *Age*: 50 years *PMH*: Hypercholesterolaemia, hypertension *DH*: Simvastatin 40 mg, ramipril 5 mg OD *FH*: Father has diabetes *Information*: You are a GP Partner. This patient had a recent blood test: HbA1C 67 mmol/l	*PC*: "*I was asked to come in to discuss my blood test results*". *HPC*: **No polydipsia/polyuria/tiredness/weight loss.** No visual problems. No problems with sensation in the feet. **Enjoys sugary cakes.** *ICE*: No concerns. Not sure why he was asked to come today. Feels fine. *O/E*: NAD

Hypothyroidism

- Under-active thyroid gland, resulting in a decreased production of thyroxine.
- Common symptoms include tiredness, weight gain, constipation, dry skin and menorrhagia.
- Treatment is by replacing the decreased thyroid hormone with a medication called levothyroxine.

Data gathering

Open questions

- *"Your recent blood test has shown that you have an underactive thyroid gland. What do you know about hypothyroidism?"*
- *"What symptoms have you been experiencing?"*

Focused/closed questions

HPC:	*"Has your weight changed recently?"*
	"Have you been more tired than usual?"
	"Have you noticed any changes with your skin or hair?"
	"Have you experienced any hoarseness?"
	"Any bowel symptoms?"
	"Any changes to your periods?"
	"Have you been feeling low in mood lately?"
FH:	Any family history of thyroid problems or other conditions?
SH:	Who lives with you at home? Smoking/alcohol/drug history? Occupation?
DH:	Do you take any regular medications?
ICE:	*"What concerns you about these symptoms?"*
Examination:	• BP.
	• Thyroid examination (see *Appendix 1*).
	• Reflexes.

Clinical management

Investigations

- Thyroid function tests.

Explanation to patient

- Thyroxine is a hormone produced by the thyroid gland in the neck. It helps to control the body's metabolism. In hypothyroidism the thyroid gland doesn't made enough thyroxine and so the body's functions slow down. It is important that this is treated to avoid complications such as heart disease from developing.
- After starting on levothyroxine you will need to have regular thyroid function blood tests to check that the level of medication is sufficient.

Management

- Levothyroxine starting dose usually 50 mcg daily (patients receive free NHS prescriptions).
- Check TFTs 1–3 monthly until stable and then annually thereafter.
- Safety net – if symptoms not improving return to GP.

Role play

Information for doctor	Additional information for role player

Patient: Mrs SO
Age: 42 years
PMH: NIDDM
DH: Metformin 500 mg TDS, gliclazide 80 mg BD
SH: Smokes 10 cigs/day, 2 units alcohol/week. Receptionist.
Information: Recent blood test:
  • serum TSH: 7 (NR: 0.35–4.94)
  • serum T$_4$: 2 (NR: 9–19)
  • serum T$_3$ 4.5 (NR: 4–8.3)
You are a salaried GP.
	PC: "*I have come in to discuss my blood test results*".
	HPC: Has been feeling more tired than usual. Thought it was likely stress at work. **Some weight gain also. No bowel symptoms. No skin changes. No increased thirst or polyuria.** No low mood. **No hoarseness.**
	ICE: Thinks she might be anaemic.
	O/E: BMI – 28. Thyroid examination – no eye changes. No palpable neck mass. Dry skin and thin hair. Slow knee reflexes.

Hyperthyroidism

- 'Overactive' thyroid gland resulting in raised levels of thyroid hormone in the bloodstream.
- Commonest cause is Graves' disease.
- Symptoms include weight loss, palpitations, tremor, restlessness and thyroid swelling.
- Management includes medication, radio-iodine treatment or surgery.

Data gathering

Open questions
- "*Can you tell me more about the symptoms you have been experiencing?*"
- "*Can you tell me more about the neck swelling you have developed?*"

Focused/closed questions

HPC: "*Have you noticed any weight loss, tremor, palpitations or diarrhoea?*"
"*Any irritability, anxiety or changes in your energy levels?*"
"*Any neck swelling or eye changes?*"

FH: Any family history of thyroid problems?

DH: Are you taking any regular medications?

SH: Alcohol/smoking/illicit drug history? Occupation? Caffeine intake?

ICE: "*What concerns you about these symptoms?*"

Examination:
- BP, pulse and cardiac examination (check for hypertension and heart arrhythmia).
- Thyroid examination (possible signs include goitre, pretibial myxoedema, lid lag, and exophthalmos).

Clinical management

Investigations
- TFTs.
- Ultrasound scan of thyroid gland if palpable thyroid mass.

Explanation to patient
- Thyroxine is a hormone made by the thyroid gland which controls the metabolism of the body.
- In hyperthyroidism there is an overactive thyroid gland which results in an increased production of thyroxine. This results in a faster metabolism.
- With treatment the outlook is good.

Management
(based on *NHS CKS*, 2013, *Hyperthyroidism*)
- Carbimazole or propylthiouracil under specialist advice only.
- Consider prescribing a beta-blocker (e.g. propranolol) if the patient has a tremor or tachycardia.
- Radio-iodine (by specialist only).
- Surgery – involves removing part of the thyroid gland.
- Follow-up – regular thyroid function tests. If symptoms worsen to return to GP.
- Admit to hospital if severe signs and symptoms of hyperthyroidism, e.g. fever, agitation, heart failure, confusion or if the patient is systemically unwell.

Role play

Information for doctor	Additional information for role player
Patient: Ms AR *Age*: 32 years *SH*: Accountant, lives with partner. No alcohol/smoking/illicit drugs. *FH*: Nil *PMH*: Migraine *DH*: Nil *Information*: No recent consultations. You are a salaried GP.	*PC*: Weight loss, tremor, palpitations. *HPC*: Palpitations and tremor for past month. Heart beat feels fast but regular. Noticed slight neck swelling. Lost 5 kg in the past month. No visual symptoms. *ICE*: **Worried about her heart.** *O/E*: HR 100, regular. Heart sounds I + II + 0. Thyroid swelling in the neck. No eye signs.

Tired all the time

- Very common presentation in general practice.
- Approximately 50% of cases will have a psychological cause.
- Only 20–30% cases will have an identifiable physical cause.
- Differential diagnoses include depression, obstructive sleep apnoea, treatment with a sedative drug, chronic fatigue syndrome, anaemia, diabetes and thyroid disease.

Data gathering

Open questions

- *"Can you tell me more about the tiredness you've been experiencing?"*
- *"What exactly do you mean by feeling tired all the time?"*

Focused/closed questions

HPC: *"When did the problem first start?"*

"Have you identified any possible triggers for the tiredness?"

"When do you feel tired?"

"Is the problem getting worse?"

"What were your previous levels of energy like, and how do they compare with the present?"

"When do you usually go to bed, and what time do you wake up?" "Any daytime napping?"

"Have you noticed any other changes, for example, passing more urine than normal, increased thirst, sleep disturbance, skin changes or bowel problems?"

"Have you had any weight loss or night sweats?" (red flags)

"Any changes in your mood?"

"Have you been feeling anxious about anything recently?"

PMH: Any significant medical problems? Any history of cancer?

DH: Are you taking any medications? Beta-blockers? Sleeping tablets?

FH: Anyone in the family with any similar problems or any illnesses that run in the family?

SH: Smoking/alcohol/illicit drugs. Daily caffeine intake?

ICE: *"Do you have any idea why you might be feeling tired all the time?"*

Examination:
- BMI.
- Check for signs of anaemia.
- Thyroid examination – if any symptoms in the history.
- PHQ-9 questionnaire – if any symptoms of depression.

Clinical management

Investigations

- Wait a month before investigating unless atypical or symptoms suggestive of a specific cause.
- Urinalysis – to check glucose.
- FBC – to check for anaemia.
- Ferritin – check in any woman of childbearing age.
- TFTs – to check for hypothyroidism.
- U&Es – to exclude any renal problems.
- CRP, ESR and monospot test for glandular fever.
- Coeliac serology – if any GI symptoms.

Explanation to patient

- Tiredness is a very common problem, and we will try to eliminate any medical cause for the tiredness, for example, anaemia or an underactive thyroid.
- The management will depend on the cause of the tiredness.

Management

- Sleep hygiene – avoid napping in the day, reduce caffeine and alcohol, increase exercise.
- If iron deficiency anaemia – ferrous sulphate.
- If hypothyroidism – start levothyroxine.
- If depression, consider self help or anti-depressants.
- Safety net – see GP again if not improving.

Role play

Information for doctor	Additional information for role player
Patient: Mr AC *Age*: 38 years *SH*: Social worker who lives with partner. *FH*: Mother and sister – depression. *PMH*: Asthma *DH*: Salbutamol 2 puffs PRN, beclomethasone 2 puffs BD *Information*: You are a GP Partner. This patient was seen by your colleague 1 week ago due to tiredness. Was sent for blood tests: • Hb 15 g/dl (NR: 13–18) • ferritin 120 ng/ml (NR: 30–400) • serum TSH 0.65 mIU/l (NR: 0.35–4.94) • serum T$_4$ 12 pmol/l (NR: 9–19) • Na 140 mmol/l (NR: 136–145) • K 4.5mmol/l (NR: 3.5–5.1) • urea 4 mmol/l (NR: 2.5–8) • creatinine 80 mmol/l (NR: 64–111)	*PC*: *"I am feeling tired all the time and have come for my blood test results".* *HPC*: Tiredness for the past few months. **Feels a bit low in mood. Stress at work.** Not sleeping very well – wakes up very early and has difficulty getting to sleep. **Concentration at work poor.** No weight changes. No bowel or urinary symptoms. Previously quite energetic. *ICE*: Worried about what is causing the tiredness. Would like a referral if no other cause is found. *O/E*: BMI 22; PHQ-9 score 16/27 (moderate–severe depression).

Chronic fatigue syndrome

- A condition involving a complex range of symptoms that includes fatigue, malaise, headaches, sleep disturbance, difficulties with concentration and muscle aches.
- Also known as ME (myalgic encephalomyelitis).
- A diagnosis should be made after excluding other possible diagnoses, and after symptoms have persisted for at least 4 months in an adult (3 months in a child).
- Usually develops between 20 and 45 years of age and is more common in females.
- Symptoms can last for years, although the outlook for young people is more optimistic.

Data gathering

Open question

- *"Can you tell me more about the fatigue you have been experiencing?"*

Focused/closed questions

HPC: *"When did your symptoms first start?"*
       "How often do you feel tired/fatigued?"
       "Does this tiredness limit the activities that you do?"
       "Is the tiredness only after exerting yourself?"
       "How would you describe your concentration?"
       "Do you have difficulty remembering things?"
       "What is your sleep pattern like?"
       "Do you suffer with any headaches or muscle pains?"
       "Have you been feeling low in mood or more anxious than normal?"
       "Any recent weight loss or breathing problems?" (red flag)

SH: Occupation? Who lives with you at home? Smoking/ alcohol/ illicit drug history? *"Have you been under a lot of stress recently?"*

ICE: *"How is this affecting your day-to-day life?"*

Examination (to exclude other causes):

- Check temperature and look for signs of anaemia.
- Lymph nodes.
- Throat.
- Abdominal examination – check for hepatomegaly or splenomegaly.
- Mental state examination (see *Appendix 3*).

Clinical management

Investigations

- Urinalysis for protein, blood and glucose.
- Blood tests for FBC, U&Es, TFTs, LFTs, ESR, CRP, random blood glucose, CK, calcium, coeliac screen.

Explanation to patient

- Chronic fatigue syndrome is a condition resulting in long term disabling tiredness. It can also cause problems with sleep, muscle pains and/or headaches.
- The cause is not known, although it may be caused by a viral infection.
- There are no tests to prove that you have chronic fatigue syndrome, and there is no specific cure. Certain treatments can ease symptoms.

Management

(based on *NICE, 2007, CG53: Chronic fatigue syndrome/Myalgic encephalomyelitis*)

- Sleep hygiene and offer relaxation techniques.

- Introduce rest periods.
- Regular well balanced diet.
- Graded exercise therapy – gradual, progressive increase in physical activity/exercise.
- Cognitive behavioural therapy.
- Offer help through occupational health services and disability services. If possible, advise flexible adjustments to work rather than stopping altogether.
- Occupational therapy or physiotherapy if required.
- Offer information about local and national self-help and support groups.
- Offer referral to specialist within 6 months of presentation if mild CFS or 3–4 months if moderate symptoms (NICE).
- Consider offering a low dose TCA for poor sleep or pain – but not if the person is already taking an SSRI (NICE).
- Regularly review management plan every 4–6 weeks and advise to return sooner if symptoms not improving or worsening.

Role play

Information for doctor	Additional information for role player
Patient: Mrs KS *Age*: 32 years *SH*: Lives with husband. Works as teacher. *PMH*: Nil *DH*: Nil *FH*: Mother has chronic fatigue syndrome. *Information*: You are a GP Registrar.	*PC*: *"I feel so weak and have no energy".* *HPC*: Six month history of tiredness. Occasional muscle aches. Concentration generally poor. Memory ok. No weight loss. Feels tired after minimal exertion. Feels low in mood but not particularly anxious. *SH*: No alcohol/smoking/illicit drugs. *ICE*: **Thinks she might have 'ME' as her mum suffers with it and has similar symptoms. Would like a sick note (has been off work for 10 days).** *O/E*: Normal examination.

Drug and alcohol problems

Alcohol abuse

- In the UK, it is estimated that 24% of adults drink in a hazardous or harmful way (*NHS Information Centre*, 2009, *Statistics on alcohol* – www.ic.nhs.uk/statistics-and-data-collections/health-and-lifestyles/alcohol).
- Alcohol dependence is defined as a cluster of behavioural, cognitive and physiological factors that typically include a strong desire to drink alcohol, and difficulties in controlling its use (DSM-IV definition by American Psychiatric Association).
- Recommended weekly alcohol consumption limits for men are 21 units and for women 14 units.
- Alcohol-related problems include Wernicke's encephalopathy, liver disease and acute and chronic pancreatitis.
- AUDIT remains the gold standard assessment tool.
- Management includes help from local alcohol services and a detoxification programme.

Data gathering

Open question
- *"Can you tell me more about your alcohol problem?"*

Focused/closed questions

HPC: *"How much alcohol are you drinking each day?"*
"Are you binge drinking or drinking on a daily basis?"
"What exactly are you drinking?"
"Why have you decided to seek help now?"
"Has anyone been concerned about your drinking?"
"Do you get annoyed at people who comment on your drinking?"
"Do you feel guilty about your drinking?"
"Do you wake up in the morning and feel the need to have a drink of alcohol?"
"Have you ever blacked out or had a fit because of your drinking?"
"Have you been feeling low in mood?"
"Do you have any abdominal pain?"
"Any problems with your balance?"
"Have you ever had any seizures?"
"Have you noticed any yellow discoloration of your skin?"

PMH: Any past problems with alcohol?

SH: Smoking//illicit drug history? Occupation? Who lives with you at home? Do you drive? *"Have you been feeling more stressed recently?"*

FH: Any FH of alcohol problems?

ICE: *"What help would you like with your drinking problem?"*

Examination:
- BP.
- Focused examination including check for tremor, jaundice, spider naevi, and abdominal examination.
- Cognitive function.
- Use formal assessment tools to assess the nature and severity of alcohol misuse. Use the AUDIT tool for identification and a routine outcome measure, and SADQ or LDQ for severity of depression. Use CIWA-Ar for severity of withdrawal.

Clinical management

Investigations
- Bloods – FBC, B_{12}, folate, LFTs, GGT.
- Liver ultrasound scan if abnormal LFTs.

Explanation to patient
- It is very important that you cut down on your drinking, as persistent drinking at harmful levels can result in damage to almost every organ or system of the body.

Management
- Advise patient to contact local alcohol services, e.g. Alcoholics Anonymous.
- Offer brief intervention CBT.
- Offer guided self help with provision of written materials.
- Consider referral for specialist assessment if the patient's AUDIT score is ≥20.
- Vitamins – vitamin B co-strong 30 mg daily, thiamine 200–300 mg daily.
- Detoxification – benzodiazepines such as chlordiazepoxide and diazepam are used in UK clinical practice for the management of alcohol-related withdrawal symptoms (*NICE*, 2011, *CG115 Alcohol-use disorders: physical complications*).
- Consider acamprosate and/or naltrexone for those who wish to abstain from alcohol.
- Nalmefene – novel therapy in alcohol management because it is initiated while the patient is still drinking. It is used to help reduce alcohol consumption in adults with alcohol dependence.
- If any symptoms/signs of delirium tremens (tremor, confusion, fits, visual hallucinations), or if at high risk of alcohol withdrawal seizures, refer urgently to hospital for medically assisted withdrawal (*NICE*, 2011, *CG115: Alcohol-use disorders: physical complications*).
- Offer social support – sick note, benefits, employment, housing, DVLA, etc.
- Regularly review every few days during period of withdrawal or abstinence and safety net – return to GP or go to A&E if any seizures, problems with withdrawal or symptoms of Wernicke's delirium tremens as described above.

Role play

Information for doctor	Additional information for role player
Patient: Mrs PP *Age*: 52 years *SH*: Recently separated from husband, lives with 2 children. Housewife. *PMH*: Nil *DH*: Nil *Information*: Last appointment was with salaried GP 6 months ago due to marital problems. You are a GP Partner.	*PC*: Drinking problem. *HPC*: Came to discuss drinking problem. Has been drinking 2 bottles of wine each night for the past couple of months since separating from husband. Concerned about her drinking and feels guilty about it. **No blackouts or seizures. Feeling a bit low also. Doesn't drive.** *SH*: No illicit drug use, non-smoker *ICE*: **Worried as husband has been physically abusive. Sister also very concerned about her drinking and wants to take the children away from her.** *O/E*: Abdominal exam NAD, BP 145/90.

Opiate addiction

- Opiate addiction is a disorder of the central nervous system that arises from continuous use of opiates.
- There is a growing problem of dependency on opiate drugs, for example, prescription drugs such as morphine and codeine and non-prescription drugs such as heroin.
- Signs of excessive opiate use include sedation, euphoria, respiratory depression, small pupils, nausea, vomiting, slurred speech and confusion.
- Abrupt or sudden withdrawal of these drugs induces a withdrawal syndrome which includes symptoms of insomnia, sweating, irritability, vomiting, depression and muscle pain.

Data gathering

Open questions
- *"Can you tell me more about your drug addiction problem?"*
- *"What is the reason for the consultation today?"*

Focused/closed questions
HPC: *"How long have you had the addiction for?"*
"Have you ever injected drugs?" "If so, have you ever shared needles?"
"Have you ever tried to get help for this problem before?" "If so, what happened?"
"Have you come today for more opiate medication or do you want help in trying to stop?"
"Do you have any problems with your sleep or your mood?"
"Any vomiting, irritability or muscle aches?" (red flags)

"Any thoughts of self harm?"
"Have you experienced any hallucinations?"
"Do you have any chest pain or shortness of breath?" (red flags)
"How is your mood?"

PMH: Have you had any previous contact with drug treatment and rehab services?

Any previous history of drug/alcohol problems?

Any past psychiatric history?

Any history of Hep B/C/HIV?

SH: Who lives with you at home? How is this problem impacting on other family members? Occupation? Finances? Smoking/alcohol?

Forensic history: Past custodial sentences, probation, community service.

ICE: *"What help would you like for your drug dependency?"*

Examination:
- Pulse, BP.
- Check for evidence of poor nutrition, dental caries, skin abscesses, needle tracks.
- Signs of acute withdrawal – sweating, watering eyes, rhinorrhoea, yawning, sneezing, dilated pupils, tremor, restlessness, etc.

Clinical management

Investigations
- ECG if concerned about heart rate/rhythm.
- Urine drug screen.
- Hep B/C, HIV testing.
- FBC, LFTs

Explanation to patient
- After prolonged opiate drug use, the nerve cells in the brain, which would otherwise produce natural painkillers (known as endorphins), cease to function normally. The body stops producing endorphins because it is receiving opiates instead. The degeneration of these nerve cells causes a physical dependency to opiate drugs.

Management
(based on *NICE CKS*, 2015, *Opioid dependence*)
- Offer information and advice on safer sex, the dangers of sharing needles and other equipment, and the risks of acquiring blood-borne viruses and other infections.
- Hepatitis A and B immunisation if IV drug user. Ensure tetanus immunisation is also up to date.
- Needle exchange programme if continuing to use IV drugs.
- Self-help/support groups – local drug services.
- Detoxification/substitution programme – methadone or buprenorphine should be offered as first line treatment in opioid detoxification.

- A report should be made to the National Drug Treatment Monitoring System when a person first starts treatment for drug misuse.
- Assess personal, social and mental health needs – housing, benefits, DVLA, etc.
- Offer CBT or psychodynamic therapy for people who have co-morbid depression and anxiety disorders (*NICE*, 2007, *CG52: Drug misuse: opioid detoxification*).
- Review patient on a weekly basis and ask them to return sooner if any new or worsening symptoms.

Role play

Information for doctor	Additional information for role player
Patient: Mr JE *Age*: 38 years *SH*: Unemployed, lives alone in a council flat. Smokes 20 cigs/day, drinks 20 units alcohol/wk. *PMH*: Nil *Information*: You are a locum GP.	*PC*: "*I would like help to get clean from drugs*". *HPC*: Currently heroin user – injects. Has been using IV drugs for the past 2 years. Doesn't share needles. Never tried to detox before. **Has had Hep B vaccine. Been tested for HIV/Hep B/C – negative.** Has difficulty sleeping. Feels low. Has financial problems also. *ICE*: Would like to start on a methadone programme. Never tried to quit before. *O/E*: Pulse and BP normal. No infected injection sites.

Appendix 1

Clinical examinations

Focused cardiovascular examination

- Expose the patient appropriately (ask permission first).
- Position the patient correctly (ideally at 45°).
- Inspection – pallor, cyanosis, scars, oedema, clubbing, JVP.
- Palpation – pulses (rate, rhythm), BP, apex beat, heaves, thrills.
- Auscultation – apex and carotid area (more detailed auscultation required if murmur heard). Listen to lung bases.

Focused respiratory examination

- Expose the patient appropriately (ask permission first).
- Position the patient at 45° ideally.
- Inspection – check hands for clubbing and peripheral cyanosis. Check tongue for pallor/cyanosis. Check respiratory rate and check chest for scars.
- Palpation – check for position of trachea and chest expansion. Check for cervical lymphadenopathy.
- Percussion – front and back of chest ideally.
- Auscultation – listen at front and back.

Focused gastrointestinal examination

- Expose the patient appropriately (ask permission first).
- Lie the patient flat if possible, with arms to the side.
- Inspection – check for jaundice, pallor, spider naevi or gynaecomastia. Check hands for clubbing, cyanosis, palmar erythema or Dupuytren's contracture. Check abdomen for distended veins or masses.
- Palpation – check for cervical lymphadenopathy. Palpate each area of the abdomen then palpate liver, spleen, kidneys and bladder (or focus depending on history).
- Percussion – liver, spleen and for shifting dullness if relevant.
- Auscultation – check for presence and quality of bowel sounds.

Neurological examination

Cranial nerves

I	Olfactory	Have you noticed any change in your sense of smell or taste?
II	Optic	Any problems with your vision? If so, check visual acuity with Snellen chart. Also check visual fields. Fundoscopy.
III	Occulomotor	Accommodation, visual movements, direct/consensual light reflex.
IV	Trochlear	As for occulomotor tests.
V	Abducens	Same as occulomotor and trochlear tests.
VI	Trigeminal	Check sensation on both sides of the face and compare (branches of trigeminal nerve).
VII	Facial	Raise eyebrows, clench teeth, blow cheeks out, close eyes tightly and stop me from opening them.
VIII	Vestibulo- cochlear	Check gross hearing by whispering in each ear. If any concerns with hearing perform Rinne's and Weber's tests.
IX	Glosso-pharyngeal	Taste sensation as above.
X	Vagal	Say 'aaaagghh' (look for deviation of the uvula).
XI	Accessory	Please can you shrug your shoulders? Check power in sternocleidomastoid muscles by moving neck side to side against resistance.
XII	Hypoglossal	Can you stick your tongue out? (check for deviation, atrophy and fasciculations).

Whispered speech test

- To make a basic assessment of a patient's hearing, you need to mask the non-test ear by blocking it with your finger, and then ask them to repeat random numbers that you speak into the test ear.
- You can start with a whisper, and if they are unable to hear this then increase the volume in incremental steps.

Rinne's test

- Strike a 512 Hz tuning fork and place the fork behind the ear, firmly on the mastoid process.
- Then hold the vibrating fork a few inches away in front of the ear.
- In a normal ear, the patient should hear the tuning fork louder in front of the ear than behind.
- If a patient has a conductive hearing loss, they will hear the bone conduction behind the ear louder than the air conduction.

Weber's test

- Strike a 512 Hz tuning fork and place the base of the fork on the patient's forehead.
- A patient with normal hearing should hear the sound equally on both sides.
- If a patient has unilateral conductive hearing loss, the sound will localise to the affected ear.
- If a patient has unilateral sensorineural loss, the sound will localise to the opposite ear.

Thyroid examination

- Hands – check pulse, check for tremor.
- Eyes – check for exophthalmos and lid lag.
- Neck – inspect, check swallowing and tongue protrusion, palpate neck for mass, percuss neck swelling, auscultate for bruits.
- Check reflexes.

Shoulder examination

- Expose both shoulders (ask permission first).
- Look – from front, side and rear inspecting for scars, erythema, muscle wasting, asymmetry, swelling and any deformity of the shoulder joint.
- Feel – check temperature, palpate bony landmarks, joint line and surrounding muscles for any tenderness, crepitus or effusions.
- Move – check active/passive movements of abduction/adduction, flexion/extension, internal/external rotation.
- Function – arms behind head and scratching back.
- Cross arm test – ask the patient to place their hand on their opposite shoulder. If gentle pressure on the joint elicits pain, this is indicative of acromioclavicular joint inflammation.
- Drop arm test – passively abduct the patient's shoulder. Then ask the patient to lower the abducted arm slowly to the waist. A rotator cuff tear can be identified if the arm drops to the side (especially beyond 90°).

Knee examination

- See www.youtube.com/watch?v=fNUGyNYVhqE to watch examination being carried out.
- Look – inspect the patient lying and standing for any scars, swelling, erythema, deformity (e.g. varus/valgus) or muscle wasting around the knee.
- Feel – palpate the medial and lateral joint line with the knee flexed. Then with the knee extended palpate the patella and the popliteal fossa. Check for effusion using a patellar tap and then check temperature on both sides.
- Move – check active/passive flexion/extension.
- Anterior drawer test – tests for stability of anterior cruciate ligament.
- Lachman's test – tests for stability of anterior cruciate ligament.
- Function – assess gait.

Elbow examination

- See www.youtube.com/watch?v=bMJjbIT3zek&NR=1&feature=fvwp to watch examination being carried out.
- Look – from front, side and back, looking at the carrying angle and for any flexion deformity, scars, swelling, rheumatoid nodules, etc.
- Feel – check temperature and palpate the olecranon and lateral/medial epicondyles for tenderness.
- Move – flexion, extension, pronation and supination (active and passive).
- Function – e.g. put hand to mouth.

Back examination

- Look – from behind inspect for deformity (lordosis/scoliosis/kyphosis), bruising, swelling, muscle wasting, asymmetry.
- Feel – check temperature, palpate spinal processes, sacro-iliac joint and para-spinal muscles for tenderness.
- Move – flexion, extension, lateral flexion, hip rotation, straight leg raise.
- Limb reflexes and sensation.
- Gait.

Diabetic foot examination

- Inspection – gait, ulcers, deformity, erythema, swelling.
- Palpation – foot pulses, temperature, capillary refill.
- Sensation – soft touch, pinprick, vibration, proprioception, temperature.
- Motor – check range of movement of foot.

Neurological motor and sensory examination
(see www.patient.co.uk for further details)

- Observation – involuntary movements, muscle symmetry, atrophy and gait.
- Tone – ask the patient to relax. Flex and extend wrists, elbows, knees and ankles. Observe for increased or decreased tone. Check for clonus also.
- Power – ask the patient to move against your resistance. Always compare one side to the other. Grade the power based on the MRC scale 0–5. Test upper and lower limbs.
- Reflexes – biceps, triceps, knee, ankle and wrist.
- Check plantar response (Babinski).
- Co-ordination – heel/shin and finger–nose test.
- Sensation – close eyes, compare symmetrical areas of the body. Check light touch first, and can continue with other modalities if any abnormalities detected.

Appendix 2

Sexual history taking

- Firstly explain that you are going to ask a few sensitive questions that are important in order to find out more about the problem.
- Ensure that the patient is relaxed and don't be judgemental.
- Privacy and assurance of confidentiality are also important.

Questions to ask

- *"When did you last have sexual intercourse?"*
- *"Was it with a regular partner or a casual partner?"*
- *"Was your partner male or female?"*
- *"Did you have vaginal sex, oral sex or anal sex?"*
- *"Did you use a condom?"*
- *"Have you had any other sexual partners in the past 3 months?"* If so, repeat the questions as above.
- *"Have you had any previous STIs?"*
- Females: *"When was your last menstrual period?" "Do you use regular contraception?" "If so, what?" "When was your last cervical smear?" "Any previous abnormal smear tests?"*
- HIV/Hep B/Hep C risk assessment: *"Have you ever paid for sex?" "Any sexual partners from high risk countries such as Thailand or sub-Saharan African countries?" "Have you or your partner ever injected drugs?" "Have you ever been vaccinated against hepatitis B?"*

Additional questions to ask those under 16 years

- *"How old is your partner?"*
- *"Was the sex consensual or did you feel coerced/forced?"*
- *"Are your parents/carer aware of your sexual activity?"*
- *"Are your parents/carer aware of your attendance here today?"*
- *"Do you feel able to tell your parents/carer?"*
- *"Have you ever been drunk or under the influence of drugs when having sexual intercourse?"*
- Any history of depression or other mental health problems?

N.B. Where children under the age of 13 report sexual activity, this should be discussed, in confidence, with a local child protection lead. Reporting to social services and the police may be appropriate but is not mandatory.

Appendix 3

Mental state examination

The following should be observed and commented on:
- **Appearance and behaviour** – patient's self care, eye contact, gait, and whether the patient is agitated, hostile or has abnormal movements.
- **Speech** – rate, volume and pressure of speech. Also note whether any incoherence, neologisms or mutism.
- **Mood** – patient's mood subjectively and objectively.
- **Thought** – content of thoughts and form (flight of ideas, thought block, etc.)
- **Perception** – any hallucinations (e.g. visual or auditory) or delusions?
- **Insight** – does the patient have any insight into their illness/mental state?

Abbreviated mental state examination

The following questions should be asked to a patient to assess cognition/memory (total score out of 10):
1. Age
2. Time
3. Address – remember 42 West Street (for recall later)
4. Year
5. Name of current location
6. Identification of two people
7. Date of birth
8. Year of World War I
9. Present monarch
10. Count out 20 down to 1
11. Recall address from earlier

Mental Capacity Act assessment

What is mental capacity?

- Mental capacity is the ability to make a decision.
- This includes the ability to make a decision that affects daily life, such as when to get up, what to wear, as well as more serious or significant decisions.
- It also refers to a person's ability to make a decision that may have legal consequences, for them or others. Examples include agreeing to have medical treatment, or making a will.
- The starting point must always be to assume that a person has the capacity to make a specific decision.

What does the Act mean by 'lack of capacity'?

- A person lacks capacity in relation to a matter if at a particular time he is unable to make a decision for himself in relation to the matter because of an impairment of, or a disturbance in, the functioning of the mind or brain. This means that a person lacks capacity if:
  - they have an impairment or disturbance (e.g. a disability, condition or trauma) that affects the way their mind or brain works, and
  - the impairment or disturbance means that they are unable to make a specific decision at the time it needs to be made (not their ability to make decisions in general).

Assessing capacity

Anyone assessing someone's capacity to make a decision for themselves should use the two-stage test of capacity.

1. Does the person have an impairment of the mind or brain, or is there some sort of disturbance affecting the way their mind or brain works? (It doesn't matter whether the impairment or disturbance is temporary or permanent.)
2. If so, does that impairment or disturbance mean that the person is unable to make the decision in question at the time it needs to be made?

Assessing ability to make a decision

1. Does the person have a general understanding of what decision they need to make and why they need to make it?
2. Does the person have a general understanding of the likely consequences of making, or not making, this decision?
3. Is the person able to understand, retain, use and weigh up the information relevant to this decision?

4. Can the person communicate their decision (by talking, using sign language or any other means)? Would the services of a professional (such as a speech and language therapist) be helpful?
5. In more complex decision making, is there a need for a more thorough assessment (perhaps by involving a doctor or other professional expert)?

The General Practitioner assessment of COGnition (GPCOG)

Patient name: _____   Date: _____

Step 1: Patient Examination

Unless specified, each question should only be asked once

Name and Address for subsequent recall test

1. *"I am going to give you a name and address. After I have said it, I want you to repeat it. Remember this name and address because I am going to ask you to tell it to me again in a few minutes: John Brown, 42 West Street, Kensington."* (Allow a maximum of 4 attempts).

	Correct	Incorrect
Time Orientation		
2. *What is the date?* (exact only)	☐	☐
Clock Drawing – use blank page		
3. *Please mark in all the numbers to indicate the hours of a clock* (correct spacing required)	☐	☐
4. *Please mark in hands to show 10 minutes past eleven o'clock* (11:10)	☐	☐
Information		
5. *Can you tell me something that happened in the news recently?* (Recently = in the last week. If a general answer is given, eg "war", "lot of rain", ask for details. Only specific answer scores).	☐	☐
Recall		
6. *What was the name and address I asked you to remember?*		
John	☐	☐
Brown	☐	☐
42	☐	☐
West (St)	☐	☐
Kensington	☐	☐

To get a total score, add the number of items answered correctly

Total correct (score out of 9)   ☐

If patient scores 9, no significant cognitive impairment and further testing not necessary
If patient scores 5–8, more information required. Proceed with Step 2, informant section.
If patient scores 0–4, cognitive impairment is indicated. Conduct standard investigations.

Step 2: Informant Interview

Date: _____

Informant's name: _____

Informant's relationship to patient, i.e. informant is the patient's: _____

These six questions ask how the patient is compared to when s/he was well, say 5–10 years ago
Compared to a few years ago:

	Yes	No	Don't know	N/A
• Does the patient have more trouble remembering things that have happened recently than s/he used to?	☐	☐	☐	
• Does he or she have more trouble recalling conversations a few days later?	☐	☐	☐	
• When speaking, does the patient have more difficulty in finding the right word or tend to use the wrong words more often?	☐	☐	☐	
• Is the patient less able to manage money and financial affairs (e.g. paying bills, budgeting)?	☐	☐	☐	☐
• Is the patient less able to manage his or her medication independently?	☐	☐	☐	☐
• Does the patient need more assistance with transport (either private or public)?	☐	☐	☐	☐

(If the patient has difficulties due only to physical problems, e.g. bad leg, tick 'no')

(To get a total score, add the number of items answered 'no', 'don't know' or 'N/A')

Total score (out of 6)   ☐

If patient scores 0–3, cognitive impairment is indicated. Conduct standard investigations.

Reproduced with permission of John Wiley and Sons, from Brodaty *et al.*, *JAGS* 2002;50:530–534.

Appendix 4

Driving and DVLA guidelines

A summary of the latest DVLA guidelines (March 2016) for some common medical conditions seen in general practice is provided below (information obtained from *DVLA at a glance guide to the current medical guidelines*, www.dft.gov.uk/dvla/medical/aag.aspx). Please refer to the website for any conditions not covered and for further guidance regarding group 2 licences.

Types of driving licence

Group 1	Group 2
Cars and motorcycles	Lorries, buses and minibuses
Valid until 70 years of age	Can usually only be issued after age 21
No upper age limit	Valid until age 45 years
Renewable every 3 years after age 70	After age 45 licence is renewable every 5 years until age 65, then renewable annually

Neurological conditions

Condition	Group 1
Epilepsy or multiple unprovoked seizures	Must not drive and must notify DVLA. If there have been no seizures for 5 years (with medication if necessary) and no other disqualifying condition, a 'Till 70' licence is usually restored.
First unprovoked epileptic seizure/isolated seizure	Must notify DVLA. 6 months off driving from date of seizure unless there are factors suggesting an unacceptably high risk of further seizure.
Single TIA	Must not drive for 1 month. May resume driving after this period if good clinical recovery. No need to routinely inform DVLA.
Multiple TIA	Driving may resume after 3 months if no further TIAs. Must notify DVLA.
Stroke	Must not drive but no need to notify the DVLA. Driving may resume after 1 month if there has been satisfactory clinical recovery. The DVLA does not need to be notified unless there is residual neurological deficit 1 month after the episode and, in particular, visual field defects or cognitive defects and impaired limb function.
Chronic neurological disorders, e.g. MS, PD	Must notify the DVLA. May drive as long as safe vehicle control is maintained at all times. Can be issued a 1, 2 or 3-year licence providing medical assessment confirms that driving ability is not impaired.

Diabetes

	Group 1	Group 2
Requires insulin	All the following criteria must be met for DVLA to license the person with insulin-treated diabetes for 1, 2 or 3 years: • Adequate awareness of hypoglycaemia • No more than 1 episode of severe hypoglycaemia in the preceding 12 months • Practises appropriate blood glucose monitoring (no more than 2 hours before the start of a journey and every 2 hours while driving) • not regarded as a likely risk to the public while driving • meets the visual standards for acuity and visual fields.	1-year licence issued if all the following standards are met: • no episode of hypoglycaemia requiring the assistance of another person in the preceding 12 months • has full awareness of hypoglycaemia • monitors blood glucose at least twice daily and at times relevant to driving (no more than 2 hours before the start of the 1st journey and every 2 hours while driving); more frequent testing may be required if for any reason there is a greater risk of hypoglycaemia, e.g. physical activity or altered meal routine • 3 months of blood glucose readings are available at annual examination by an independent consultant diabetologist • can demonstrate an understanding of the risks of hypoglycaemia
Diet or tablet controlled	No need to inform DVLA unless complications or insulin needed.	May drive but must notify the DVLA. All the following criteria must be met for the DVLA to issue a licence for 1, 2 or 3 years: • no episode of severe hypoglycaemia in the last 12 months • full awareness of hypoglycaemia • regular self-monitoring of blood glucose – at least twice daily and at times relevant to driving • demonstrates an understanding of the risks of hypoglycaemia • has no disqualifying complications of diabetes that mean a licence will be refused or revoked, such as a visual field defect.

Cardiac conditions

Condition	Group 1
Acute coronary syndromes	Must not drive but need not notify the DVLA. Driving may resume 1 week after successful coronary angioplasty and if no other urgent revascularisation planned, LV ejection fraction is at least 40% and if no other disqualifying condition. If no successful coronary angioplasty, driving may resume only after 4 weeks from acute event.
Angina	Must not drive when symptoms occur at rest, with emotion or at the wheel. Driving may resume after satisfactory symptom control. Need not notify the DVLA.
Angioplasty (elective)	Driving must cease for at least 1 week.
CABG	Driving must cease for at least 4 weeks. No need to notify DVLA.
Arrhythmias likely to cause incapacity	Must not drive and may need to notify the DVLA. Driving may resume without DVLA notification only after the underlying cause has been identified and the arrhythmia is controlled for at least 4 weeks.

Respiratory conditions

Condition	Group 1
Obstructive sleep apnoea	Stop driving until satisfactory control of symptoms, confirmed by medical review.

Psychiatric conditions and alcohol use

Condition	Group 1
Dementia	May be able to drive but must notify the DVLA. It is difficult to assess driving ability in people with dementia. The DVLA acknowledges that there are varied presentations and rates of progression, and the decision on licensing is usually based on medical reports.
Acute psychotic disorder	Driving must cease during the acute episode and the DVLA must be notified. Re-licensing can be considered when well for at least 3 months and compliant with treatment, confirmed by specialist report.
Alcohol misuse	Cease driving until 6 months of controlled drinking/abstinence with normal blood markers. Must notify the DVLA.
Alcohol dependence	Licence may be returned after 1 year of abstinence and normal blood markers.

Appendix 5

When to suspect child maltreatment

Based on *NICE, 2009, CG89: When to suspect child maltreatment*

Child maltreatment

- Includes physical, emotional and sexual abuse, neglect, and fabricated or induced illness.
- The level of concern of child maltreatment can be divided into two main categories:
    1. **Consider** – maltreatment is one possible explanation for the alerting feature or is included in the differential diagnosis.
    2. **Suspect** – serious level of concern about the possibility of child maltreatment but not proof of it.

Risk factors for child maltreatment

- Previous history of child abuse in the family.
- Domestic violence (see *Appendix 7*).
- Mental illness, physical illness or disability in the carers.
- Drug or alcohol misuse in the carer.
- Housing or financial problems.
- Disability in the child.
- Single parents, especially if unsupported.

Assessment

History

- Use open and non-judgemental questions, e.g. *"What happened?"* rather than leading questions, e.g. *"Did you hit her?"*.
- Take a history directly from the child if it is in their best interests – be alert to the fact that they may not show any outward signs of abuse.
- If using an interpreter this should ideally not be a family member.
- Listen carefully, taking into account symptoms, signs, information disclosed, child's appearance, behaviour and interaction between the child and carer.
- Record accurately what is said and observed, by whom, and why you are concerned.

- If you are considering or suspecting child abuse think about your level of concern, discuss with colleagues, refer and/or seek more information.

Examination

- Obtain consent for a physical examination specifically for child protection purposes. In an emergency, it may be in the child's best interests to have this examination without explicit consent (remember to document the reasons).
- Document all findings and record any examination findings/signs on a body map.

Possible signs and symptoms of child maltreatment

- Injuries which are multiple, frequent, or of different ages.
- Injuries which are not consistent with the history or developmental age of the child, e.g. fractures in infants.
- No explanation for the injuries, or a child's story differing from that of the carers.
- Delayed presentation.
- Unexplained denial or aggression.
- Unexplained anxiety, fearfulness or withdrawal from the child.
- Unusual reluctance to undress or fear of physical contact during medical assessment.
- Frozen watchfulness.
- Bruising in the shape of a hand, ligature, teeth mark, etc.
- Petechiae not caused by a medical condition – may be due to shaking.
- Burns showing the shape of an implement, e.g. cigarette or iron.
- Scald with clear demarcation and symmetrical.
- Fracture in a baby too young to walk or crawl.
- Multiple fractures in different stages of healing.
- Retinal haemorrhages without major confirmed accidental trauma or medical explanation.
- Delayed development (could indicate emotional abuse).
- Carers repeatedly humiliating the child.
- Child's unexplained fear of a known adult.
- Secondary enuresis or faecal soiling.
- Genital symptoms/signs – dysuria, soreness, bleeding or discharge, anal fissure, sexually transmitted infection without clear evidence of vertical transmission.
- Failure to thrive.
- Poor hygiene and unkempt.
- Frequent school absence.

Investigations

- Blood tests – FBC, clotting screen (if suspecting child abuse, these investigations should not delay referral).
- Other investigations, e.g. skeletal survey or CT head should only be done after referring to secondary care.

Management in primary care

- If you think a child may be at risk, discuss your concerns with colleagues, e.g. health visitor, nurse, lead GP for child protection or with social services.
- Document all your concerns, discussions and decisions.
- After discussion, if you still have concerns refer the child and family to social services.
- If you think the child is at immediate risk of serious harm, refer immediately to the police and social services.
- If the child requires referral/admission to hospital, refer to a paediatrician and ensure they are aware of your concerns.
- Always remember the child's welfare is paramount and their best interests override other considerations such as confidentiality and consent.
- Remember other children in the household – are they at risk?
- Ensure that the child and family have follow-on care.
- Housekeeping – remember to look after yourself as you may also need support.

Appendix 6

Discussion following myocardial infarction

Recovery

- Recovering from a heart attack can take several months, and the two most important aims are to gradually restore your physical fitness so you can resume normal activities and to reduce your risk of another heart attack.
- A person's cardiac rehabilitation programme will begin whilst in hospital, and patients will usually be invited back for another session within 10 days of leaving hospital.
- Once you return home, it is usually recommended that you rest and only do light activities such as walking up and down the stairs a few times a day or taking a short walk.

Work

- In terms of returning to work, it obviously will depend on your health, the state of your heart and the kind of work that you do. If your job involves light duties you may be able to return in as little as two weeks. If you have a heavy manual job, it may be several months before you can return to work.

Sex

- According to the British Heart Foundation, you are usually able to start having sex again once you feel well enough, usually about four to six weeks after having a heart attack. Having sex will not put you at further risk of having another heart attack.
- Following a heart attack, about one in three men will have erectile dysfunction. This is most commonly due to the emotional stress associated with having a heart attack, but can also be a side effect of beta-blockers.

Driving

- Following an MI you must not drive but you need not notify the DVLA for class 1 vehicles. If you drive a lorry or bus you must notify the DVLA.
- Driving may resume 1 week after successful coronary angioplasty. If no successful coronary angioplasty, driving may resume after 4 weeks provided there are no other disqualifying conditions.

Appendix 7

Domestic violence

- Domestic violence and abuse is a complex issue that needs sensitive handling by all healthcare professionals.
- It can be linked to chronic health problems, PTSD, depression, anxiety and substance misuse.
- Don't forget that men can be victims too.
- Different types include partner abuse amongst adults or young people, abuse between parents, honour-based violence and forced marriage, abuse of older people and abuse of parents by children.

Summary of *NICE* guidance 2014

- Have a high index of suspicion:
  - repeat attenders, chronic health problems, PTSD, depression, anxiety, substance abuse.
- Have clear and good lines of communication when people are considered at risk.
- Create an environment to disclose abuse:
  - posters on waiting room walls
  - leaflets in consulting rooms
  - ensure front line staff, including reception and admin teams, are aware of the referral processes and local support networks.
- Ensure you ask about abuse if suspected:
  - tailor support to each individual. Have a card/leaflet to hand out with support networks information
  - prioritise patient safety
  - refer children to social services if domestic violence is suspected or disclosed.

Tips for a domestic violence/abuse consultation

- Do not ask about domestic violence in the presence of another family member.
- Do not 'force' a disclosure; this may take years, but just asking is helpful for victims.
- Start with non-judgemental open questions:
  - *"Are there any problems at home?"*
  - *"Sometimes people who attend here often have experienced abuse at home – might that be happening to you?"*
- Move on to more direct questions:
  - *"Are you afraid of your partner/relative?"*
  - *"Have they hurt you, now or in the past?"*

- The **HARK** questions have been developed and validated in primary care:
  - Does your partner **h**umiliate or **h**it you?
  - Are you ever **a**fraid of your partner?
  - Has your partner ever **r**aped you?
  - Has your partner ever **k**icked or physically hurt you?
- Acknowledge admission of abuse:
  - *"Thank you for trusting us to tell us"*
  - *"You are not alone"*
  - *"Help is available"*
- Provide details of local agencies.
- Consider child protection – guidelines suggest a child protection referral in all cases where a child under 12 years is in the household.
- Assess safety and risk of immediate harm:
  - *"Are you safe to go home?"* Discuss contacting police.
- Document any injuries clearly, including taking photographs.